Y0-BUP-299

Malignant Solid Tumors in Children
A Review

Malignant Solid Tumors
in Children
A Review

Wataru W. Sutow, M.D.

Pediatrician and Professor of Pediatrics
The University of Texas System Cancer Center,
M. D. Anderson Hospital and Tumor Institute,
Houston, Texas

Raven Press ■ New York

Raven Press, 1140 Avenue of the Americas, New York, New York 10036

Made in the United States of America

Library of Congress Cataloging in Publication Data

Sutow, Wataru Walter, 1912–
  Malignant solid tumors in children.

  Includes bibliographical references and index.
  1.   Tumors in children.   I.   Title.   [DNLM:
1.   Neoplasms—In infancy and childhood.   QZ200
S967m]
RC281.C4S99   618.92'994   77–94670
ISBN 0–89004–299–3

Preface

This volume provides a review of several selected aspects of childhood malignant solid tumors. I have attempted to look beyond the customary tables and graphs and to use data compiled from a number of sources to provide meaningful and usable perspectives. Such perspectives cover the practical aspects of management and also some philosophical and ethical considerations that may be involved. It is hoped that this broad approach will aid in the formulation of treatment plans and in the interpretations of clinical developments.

Although significant progress has been made in the control of Wilms' tumor, osteosarcoma, and a few other tumor types, frustrating questions about effective therapy for such tumors as neuroblastoma, Ewing's sarcoma and brain tumors, remain unanswered. It is anticipated that a careful assessment of the principles and strategies used in the successful control of some cancers will result in purposeful extrapolation of similar considerations to the problem areas.

The attitudes toward and the evaluation of progress in pediatric oncology, as expressed here, reflect author bias. In particular, I am prejudiced against the overuse of detailed "therapeutic recipes," and believe that published information should be considered only as guidelines for treatment decisions that will vary with the clinical circumstances in individual patients.

The discussions in this book are limited to tumor studies with which I have had the most direct personal experience during my association, since 1954, with the University of Texas System Cancer Center M.D. Anderson Hospital and Tumor Institute.

This volume will be of interest to all health professionals concerned with the delivery of total care to the children with malignant solid tumors.

Wataru W. Sutow, M.D.

Contents

1

General Considerations

STATISTICS OF CHILDHOOD CANCER

Incidence

Two recent publications provide more precise estimates of the incidence of cancer in children than have been available before. Young and Miller (96) summarized the pediatric aspects of the Third National Cancer Survey (15). The Survey, designed by the Biometry Branch of the National Cancer Institute, was conducted over a 3-year period, from 1969 to 1971, which overlapped the National Census of 1970. Thus population-based calculations of incidence rates in the United States have been derived.

Table 1 gives a condensed tabulation of the data from Young and Miller (96) to indicate the incidence rates for the tumor categories discussed in this book. This table also includes, for comparative purposes, the updated incidence figures from the Manchester Children's Tumour Registry (Great Britain) (42).

The second publication (95) was distributed by the American Cancer Society in September, 1978. These incidence data were derived for the years 1973 to 1976 from the Surveillance, Epidemiology, and End Results (SEER) program of the National Cancer Institute. The survey used 10 population-based registries. The SEER program, however, covered geographic areas different from the Third National Cancer Survey. Therefore, direct comparisons of estimates derived from the two surveys would be hazardous.

Based on the data from the SEER Program, the number of new cancers among children under 15 for the United States in 1978 is shown in Table 2.

TABLE 1. *Incidence of malignant neoplasms per million population per year in children under 15 years of age*[a]

Site	White	Black	Manchester Tumour Registry[b]
All cancer	124.5	97.8	91
Leukemia	42.1	24.3	32
Lymphoma	13.2	13.9	7
CNS	23.9	23.9	19
SNS	9.6	7.0	7
Retinoblastoma	3.4	3.0	3
Kidney	7.8	7.8	5
Liver	1.9	0.4	—
Bone	5.6	4.8	—
Gonads	2.2	2.6	—
Soft tissue	8.4	3.9	—
Miscellaneous	6.4	6.1	18

[a] Based on Third National Cancer Survey, 1969–1971 (96).
[b] From Leck (42).

TABLE 2. *Estimates of new cancers in children under age 15 in the United States in 1978*[a]

Site	No. of new cases	Percentage of new cases
All sites	6,100	100.0
Leukemias	1,875	30.7
CNS	1,100	18.0
Lymphomas	800	13.1
SNS	475	7.8
Soft tissues	400	6.6
Kidney	350	5.7
Bone	300	4.9
Eye	200	3.3
Other sites	600	9.8

[a] Based on SEER program data (95).

Additional perspectives regarding demographic aspects of childhood cancer can be obtained from inspection of the SEER program data. Thus the relative incidences of major forms of childhood cancer can be calculated by 5-year age groups for each sex (as shown in Tables 3 and 4). When solid tumors are considered as a whole (excluding leukemias and lymphomas), the relative frequencies of the major solid tumors are as indicated in Table 5. Table 6 compares incidences of various solid tumor types between the sexes, based on data from Young and Miller (96).

Tables 1 to 6 permit observations regarding the apparent patterns of cancer occurrence among children in the United States:

1. Lymphomas and bone tumors increase in relative frequency (as well as in incidence rates) with increasing age in both sexes. A marked increase of miscellaneous tumors occurs in the 10–14 age group.

TABLE 3. *Relative incidence of major forms of childhood cancer for males[a]*

	Relative incidence (%) by 5-year age groups		
Site	0–4	5–9	10–14
All sites	100.0	100.0	100.0
Leukemia	39.3	31.2	24.3
CNS	12.4	24.8	17.3
Lymphoma	5.2	19.6	24.9
SNS	16.1	2.2	0.7
Soft tissues	5.4	8.2	7.9
Kidney	7.5	4.3	0.3
Bone	0.7	2.8	13.5
Eye	5.6	1.4	0.3
Other sites	7.7	5.3	11.0
Rate for all cancers[b]	187.2	107.0	106.8

[a] Based on data from SEER program (95).
[b] Per million population per year.

TABLE 4. *Relative incidence of major forms of childhood cancer for females*[a]

Site	Relative incidence (%) by 5-year age groups		
	0–4	5–9	10–14
All sites	100.0	100.0	100.0
Leukemia	34.7	36.1	18.1
CNS	14.0	26.1	20.1
Lymphoma	4.2	7.1	19.3
SNS	14.3	5.0	2.3
Soft tissues	4.2	8.8	6.8
Kidney	12.8	6.7	2.6
Bone	0.8	3.3	8.7
Eye	7.9	—	0.3
Other sites	7.2	7.1	21.8
Rate for all cancers[b]	142.6	76.5	103.9

[a] Based on data from SEER program (95).
[b] Per million population per year.

TABLE 5. *Relative frequency of malignant solid tumors in children*[a]

Site[b]	Relative frequency (%)	
	White	Black
All solid tumors	100.0	100.0
CNS	34.5	40.2
SNS	13.9	11.8
Soft tissues	12.1	6.6
Kidney	11.3	13.1
Bone	8.1	8.1
Eye	4.9	5.0
Miscellaneous	15.2	15.3

[a] Based on tabulations of Young and Miller (96).
[b] Leukemias and lymphomas have been excluded from calculations.

TABLE 6. *Comparison of incidence of major forms of childhood cancer between sexes*[a]

Site	M:F ratio by 5-year age groups		
	0–4	5–9	10–14
All sites	1.31	1.40	1.03
Leukemias	1.49	1.21	1.38
CNS	1.16	1.33	0.89
Lymphomas	1.62	3.89	1.32
SNS	1.48	0.63	0.33
Soft tissues	1.68	1.31	1.18
Kidney	0.77	0.90	0.11
Bone	1.18	1.20	1.60
Eye	0.93	—	—
Other sites	1.41	1.06	0.52

[a] Based on tabulations from SEER program (95).

2. Neoplasms of kidney, eye, and sympathetic nervous system (SNS), as well as leukemias, decrease in relative frequency (and in incidence) with increasing age. Of these tumors, eye cancer (almost entirely retinoblastoma) is nearly limited to the 0–4 age group. Tumors of the kidney (presumably mostly Wilms' tumor) and the SNS (presumably mostly neuroblastoma) are heavily concentrated in the youngest age group.

3. Tumors of the central nervous system (CNS) and soft tissue tumors seem to peak in the 5–9 age group.

4. Total incidence rate (for all sites) per 1,000,000 population is highest in the 0–4 age group for both sexes, being higher in males than females. In the females, the total incidence drops in the 5–9 age group but rises again in the 10–14 age group. The latter rise appears to be caused by increased incidence of lymphomas and miscellaneous cancers in the older female children.

5. In practically all tumor categories and in comparable age groups, the incidence figures are higher for males compared

to females (Table 6). A prominent exception is the higher incidence rate for miscellaneous tumors among females in the 10–14 age group. It is interesting to note a definite female preponderance of kidney tumors in all age groups and a suggestive female preponderance of SNS tumors in the 5–14 age group. Tabulations of published data have shown that among Wilms' tumor patients, boys outnumber girls (8,31,84). The male/female (M:F) ratio in neuroblastoma from compiled data was reported to be 1.1 (31). Therefore, manipulations of data of this type for comparisons, which can be done facilely, must be approached with maximum caution.

Mortality from Childhood Cancer

Cancer remains a major medical problem as the leading cause of death (next to accidents) in children over the age of 3 years (93). Below that age, other medical causes, such as major cardiovascular diseases, infectious diseases, and congenital anomalies, account for most of the deaths.

Under the age of 5 years, cancer as the cause of death increases progressively from 0.3% of all deaths in infants to 12.6% of all deaths during the fourth year of age (Table 7). Over the age

TABLE 7. *Childhood deaths under 5 years of age in the United States in 1975[a]*

Age (years)	Total no. of deaths from all causes	Percent dying from cancer
Under 1	50,525	0.3
1	3,272	4.0
2	2,253	7.4
3	1,822	10.8
4	1,713	12.6

[a] From Vital Statistics (93).

TABLE 8. *Childhood deaths by age and cause in the United States in 1975[a]*

Age (years)	Total no. of deaths from all causes	Percent dying from cancer	Percent dying from accidents[b]
Under 1	50,525	0.3	—
Under 5	59,585	1.4	9.1
5–9	6,185	15.0	51.2
10–14	7,294	12.0	57.6
15–19	21,267	5.9	73.5

[a] From Vital Statistics (93).
[b] Includes also homicides and suicides.

of 5 years, accidents (including homicides and suicides) account for more than half of all deaths (Table 8). The relative cancer mortality reaches a peak in the 5–9 age group, accounting for 15% of all deaths.

Mortality calculations for specific cancers cannot be derived satisfactorily from national mortality tables. Rapidly changing survival rates resulting from increasingly effective therapy together with lack of simultaneously determined incidence figures do not provide sufficiently precise mortality rates for specific histopathologic entities. In this volume, more accurate mortality rates are indicated in the discussions of specific tumors.

NATURE OF MALIGNANT SOLID TUMORS OF CHILDHOOD

Comparison of Adult and Childhood Cancers

For 1978, the estimate of new cancers in children through 14 years of age was 6,100 (95) (see Table 2). For the entire United States population of all ages, it was estimated that in 1978 there would be 700,000 new cases of cancer (1). (This estimate excluded 40,000 new cases of carcinoma *in situ* of cervix and 300,000 cases of nonmelanoma skin cancers.) For many calculations, therefore, the minute fraction (less than 1%) of the total cancer population that constitutes children becomes overwhelmed by the proportionately massive numbers of adult cases. At the time of the Third National Cancer Survey (1969–1971) (15), 29% of the population of the United States were under 15 years of age. Therefore, more than 99% of all cancers occur in 71% of the population and 1% in 29% of the population.

The distribution of histopathologic categories of cancer in children differs strikingly from the relative frequencies of the same categories of cancer in adults. Tabulations of involvement of specific anatomic organs may provide incomplete information, since the same organ may give rise to different histopathologic entities in different age groups. For example, practically all malignant neoplasms of the kidney in children represent Wilms' tumor. In contrast, Wilms' tumor is uncommon in adults; only about 5% of all cases occur in patients over 8 years of age and less than 2% in patients over 16 years of age (8,32,84). In adults, the primary malignant tumor of the kidney is renal carcinoma, which is rare in children. During a 25-year period when 1,054 cases of renal carcinoma were seen at M.D. Anderson Hospital, 0.4% were under the age of 10 years, and 0.8% were under the age of 20 years (88).

To provide a perspective of relative frequencies of cancer categories among children compared to adults, Table 9 was derived from the data published from the Third National Cancer Survey (15). (In the preparation of the various tables for this chapter, several different sources have been utilized. The reader is cautioned to keep in mind the derivation of the data and the purpose of the individual tables.)

From inspection of Table 9, it is immediately obvious that major forms of cancer differ drastically between children and adults. The carcinomas and adenocarcinomas (involving oropharynx, digestive organs, breast, respiratory organs, genital organs, urinary organs), which account for more than 80% of adult can-

TABLE 9. *Relative frequencies of cancer categories in adults and children*

Category	Percent of all cancers[a]	
	Children under 15	Age 15 and over
Leukemia	32.5	2.9
Lymphoma	10.4	3.2
Brain and nervous system	21.1	1.4
Eye	3.3	0.2
Bone	4.7	0.2
Soft tissues	4.3	0.7
Kidney and renal pelvis	7.2	2.0
Digestive system	3.6	25.4
Respiratory system	1.8	15.2
Genital system	2.6	19.4
Urinary system[b]	0.4	4.5
Breast	—	13.6
Other	8.1	11.3

[a] Data from the Third National Cancer Survey (15).
[b] Kidney and renal pelvis are listed separately.

cer, total less than 10% of childhood cancer. Leukemias and lymphomas constitute about 5% and brain and nervous system tumors, 1.4% of adult cancer. In sharp contrast, leukemia and lymphoma account for 43% of childhood cancer and brain tumors, another 21%. Sarcomas and embryonal tumors, which make up another significant part of childhood malignancies (about 20%), contribute insignificantly (less than 1.5%) to the adult cancer statistics.

In the summary tabulations from the Third National Cancer Survey (15), the separation of neuroblastoma data from "other nervous system tumors" is difficult. The section providing histopathology data does not show the age breakdown. Among the microscopically confirmed diagnosis group,[1] neuroblastoma accounted for 0.06% of cancer cases for all ages combined.

---

[1] Neuroblastoma data were considered to be those coded as no. 9503 using the Manual of Tumor Nomenclature & Coding system, 1968 edition (2).

Etiologic Considerations

No meaningful discussion of etiology can be attempted in any single volume or by any one individual. It is the intent of these few short paragraphs to alert the clinician to "think etiologically at the bedside," as Miller (57,58) has graphically phrased it. Miller makes the point that clinical observations can provide clues that can be derived only from patients. A striking example of this perspicacious achievement was the observation that "Wilms' tumor occurs in a constellation of four growth excesses, namely, malignant neoplasia, hamartoma, congenital hemihypertrophy, and visceral cytomegaly syndrome" (57,58).

Answers to questions regarding causes and the fundamental biologic behavior of cancers should facilitate the cure of more types of cancer and possibly the prevention of some. To the clinician, however, there are immediate and practical applications of these investigative findings. They relate to the recognition of the population at risk for any given type of cancer (23) and the early cancer detection in the high-risk group (79).

Examples of high-risk correlations, that is, apparent increases in risk of cancer, are: chromosomal abnormality and leukemias, chromosomal abnormality and retinoblastoma, inborn immunologic abnormality and lymphoma, environmental exposure to carcinogenic factors (radiation and induced immunosuppression), chromosome abnormality and gonadoblastoma, and familial cancer (22,44,59,64,81,82).

A number of recent publications are available which cover various etiologic aspects of cancer. The proceedings of the conference on "Persons at High Risk of Cancer: An Approach to Cancer Etiology and Control" (23) provide a good perspective of the current status of knowledge in that area. The book entitled *Genetics of Human Cancer* (64) covers various genetic aspects related to pediatric cancer. Genetic considerations are further outlined in a subsequent section, but discussions have been published in a number of readily available sources (22,64,81). Proceedings of the International Workshop on Multiple Primary

TABLE 10. *Causation of childhood cancer by environmental factors*

Carcinogen	Cancer	Refs.
Ionizing radiation	Leukemias	30,43,54
	Osteosarcoma	30,35,43,52,54,61
	Thyroid cancer	13,30,43,51,54,61, 62,72,80
	Sarcomas	30,35,43,54
	Skin cancer	30,43,54
	Breast cancer	30,43,54,61
	Brain tumor	30,43,54,61
Androgenic-anabolic steroids	Hepatocellular carcinoma	33,53
Asbestos	Mesothelioma of pleura	3
Stilbestrol	Clear cell carcinoma of vagina/cervix	67,74
Vinyl chloride	Angiosarcoma	91

Cancers (71) and Conference on Cancer Epidemiology and the Clinician (70) give further pertinent information.

Examples of cancer caused by environmental factors, for obvious reasons, become widely publicized (30,56,59). A voluminous literature exists with respect to each known (or even suspected) factor (44,59). Table 10 indicates some of these carcinogenic environmental factors and the cancers that have resulted; only a few recent references are listed. In these cases, the latent time generally required for the development of tumor puts the patient into adult age groups and out of pediatric oncology for diagnosis and clinical management.

Genetic Considerations

Mulvihill (63) has divided the genetic factors in human oncogenesis into three groups: chromosomal, single-gene locus, and polygenic. The application of sophisticated techniques, such as banding, as well as computer techniques in karyotyping have identified specific chromosome markers [for example, in acute myelogenous leukemia, in the Wilms' tumor-aniridia syndrome, and in retinoblastoma 13 q- syndrome (81,82)].

Strong (82) has reviewed the evidence that points to cancer being "a genetic disease at the cellular level." Retinoblastoma has been utilized as a model for the study of genetic aspects of childhood cancer. From these data, Knudson (37,38) developed the two mutational step ("hit") theory and postulated the occurrence of retinoblastoma in both a hereditary and nonhereditary pattern. Subsequently, similar approaches were applied to the genetic study of other tumors, notably Wilms' tumor (39) and neuroblastoma (40).

Strong (81,82) has succinctly summarized the concept of childhood cancers occurring in both a hereditary (prezygotic) and a nonhereditary (postzygotic) form. The characteristics of the hereditary form are "autosomal dominant inheritance (once expressed), a familial pattern of affected siblings or cousins, and a predisposition to multiple primary tumors of the same or associated sites." The clinical importance of any of these "markers" translates into the probability of "transmitting a tumor predisposition to subsequent offspring as well as the risk of subsequent tumors in the affected gene carrier" (81,82).

Fraumeni (22) has considered "hereditary syndromes" (diseases of single-gene origin predisposing to cancer) under hereditary neoplasms in which the gene defect is expressed as tumor and the preneoplastic state in which a precursor lesion exists. The latter group has been further subdivided into four categories: dominantly inherited hamartomatous syndromes, recessively inherited genodermatoses, chromosome breakage disorders (chromosome fragility), and immune deficiency syndromes.

Because of steadily improving survival rates in childhood cancer, genetic considerations are becoming increasingly more important in pediatric oncology. Information and counseling are sought by the survivors and relatives in regard to the role of genetic predisposition in (a) the cause of cancer, (b) the risk of subsequent cancer in the surviving patient, (c) the risk of cancer in the offspring of survivors, and (d) the risk of cancer among relatives

(20). The calculations of risk estimates are complex, and expert genetic counseling now requires specialized knowledge. It is highly desirable that a professional with a sound background in genetics be a member of the oncology team. Examples of published estimates of risk of tumor, when available, have been incorporated in the chapters on specific tumors.

Fraumeni (22,24) has commented on "familial cancer," a risk "derived empirically from large-scale statistical survey." This risk is separated from the familial patterns of hereditary neoplastic syndromes. Statistical studies have shown "site-specific aggregations" and "multiple cancer syndromes." While methodologic questions may arise with respect to the derivation of risk statistics, it is stated that "first-degree relatives have a greater frequency of cancer of the same site, but not cancers in general" (22), being four-fold or greater for leukemia, brain tumors, and soft tissue sarcomas (22). The occurrence of cancers of dissimilar cell types in family constellations has popularized the concept of "cancer families" (24,48). In one report, rhabdomyosarcomas were observed to aggregate in siblings and to be associated with a high frequency of breast cancer in patients and their relatives (46,48). Implications of findings such as these for genetic counseling are obvious (20,22,24,48,55).

The statistical documentation that "persons who develop cancer appear to be at greater risk for the development of a second malignant neoplasm" (54) at a rate of 2 to 11% has at least two clinical implications. One is the effect on the patient and his management. A second and equally important consideration is the role of therapy in the genesis of the second cancer. Radiation-induced second malignant neoplasms are well-known (43,54). The carcinogenic hazards of cancer chemotherapeutic agents in man (4,9,94) are less well defined, although increased risk of new cancers has been suggested in patients intensively treated for Hodgkin disease. Actual patient data from multigenerational studies and long-term follow-up evaluations (20,45) only recently are becoming available in reasonably sufficient quantities to permit clinical testing of some of the hypotheses.

The genetic considerations have expanded the responsibilities of the physician in making not only the clinical diagnosis of cancer but also, to the degree possible, an etiologic diagnosis. The absolute requirement of these types of knowledge in genetic counseling is apparent. The development of effective treatment regimens for childhood cancer has been accompanied by a concomitant growth in the demand for pertinent and competent genetic counseling (47,82).

STRATEGY AND TACTICS OF CANCER THERAPY

The improving prognosis in children with nonmetastatic Wilms' tumor (16,17,87), rhabdomyosarcoma (49,50), osteosarcoma (25,27,60,85), and Ewing's sarcoma (66,68,76,77), as well as increasingly successful retrieval of patients with postmetastatic Wilms' tumor (89) and osteosarcoma (90), provide clear evidence that effective therapy regimens have been developed and utilized in pediatric oncology.

This section simply lists some of the developments that have contributed to the successful results. The general principles and overall strategy are discussed more fully in a later chapter covering the subject of multimodal therapy. The actual details of the implementation of the tactics are provided, where applicable, in the chapters on specific cancers.

The significant approaches to therapy that have been developed and successfully field tested in childhood solid tumors (86) include the following:

1. Use of drugs in combination.
2. Evaluation of new drugs and new combinations.
3. Modification of dose and schedule of drugs to provide more intensive and effective therapy.
4. Better understanding of the biologic behavior of specific cancers.
5. Identification of prognostic factors.
6. Development of effective multidisciplinary strategy of therapy and improvement in the attitudes of physicians.

7. Expanded utilization of adjuvant chemotherapy.
8. Better control of metastatic disease.
9. Concept of treating the whole child (and not just the tumor).

Some of the day-to-day, step-by-step general guidelines in the management of the child with cancer are indicated below (86):

1. The general clinical status of the patient is evaluated with particular attention to the patient's probable ability to tolerate various procedures.
2. A careful, systematic assessment of the extent of the disease (staging) is made.
3. A plan of approach, including time and site of biopsy, is agreed upon by the cancer management team.
4. The diagnosis is established and is discussed by the pathologist, particularly in reference to presence or absence of favorable/unfavorable patient characteristics (prognostic factors).
5. The pathologist and the surgeon confirm the stage of the disease in the patient.
6. Treatment is instituted in the sequence and intensity determined by the management team.
7. The progress of treatment, side effects of therapy, and results are monitored systematically and regularly, generally by the oncologist.
8. Rehabilitation procedures are instituted under collaboration of a physiatrist.
9. Long-term follow-up evaluations are continued with respect to disease activity as well as late effects of therapy.

CONCEPTS OF PROGNOSIS

Period of Risk

The period of risk has been defined as the period of time after treatment during which evidence of failure of treatment becomes apparent. Conversely, relapse after this risk period rarely occurs, and the patient may be considered "cured." On the basis of compiled past clinical experiences, models have been proposed to predict this period of risk of relapse (recurrence/metastases) after therapy.

More than two decades ago, the "Collins' rule" defined the period of risk as that duration of time after treatment equal to the patient's age plus 9 months (gestation) (11,12). The hypothesis assumed that the rate of tumor growth (doubling time) remained comparable before and after treatment and that the tumor growth could have started as early as conception. If tumor regrowth started immediately after treatment, the tumor should reach the same size as that attained at diagnosis over a period of time equal to or less than the interval between conception and diagnosis (11,12).

The concept was derived from retrospective study of survival among children with Wilms' tumor (11,12). Subsequently, it was reported that the clinical courses of neuroblastoma and rhabdomyosarcoma (childhood tumors occurring with sufficient frequency and with meaningful cure rates to permit analyses of this type) conformed closely to predictions (36).

From the practical point of view, Collins' rule, if truly valid, was readily applicable to young children 4 or 5 years of age and under. For older children, however, the duration of time needed for observation became increasingly ponderous. Consequently, a "2-year rule" was proposed, based on observations that in childhood solid tumors, the rate of growth is so rapid that treatment failures can be readily identified during a period of 2 years after therapy (69). This type of reasoning conforms in concept to the 5- and 10-year survival used traditionally in discussions of cure among adult patients.

In neuroblastoma, a period even shorter than 2 years has been suggested as adequate follow-up to select out practically all treatment failures (18,28).

Statistical Considerations

Because of increasingly effective treatment programs, survival in pediatric cancer is steadily improving, although the rate and magnitude of improvement vary from tumor to tumor. These changes have necessitated new, dynamic approaches to the assessment of prognosis not only for specific tumors but also from therapeutic epoch to therapeutic epoch. Thus biostatisticians, with their knowledge of quantitative methods of estimating survival time, have become essential staff members at comprehensive cancer centers (7,78). The impact of biostatistical methodology in clinical research has also spawned, for the clinicians, a relatively unfamiliar terminology with important connotations.

Life table methods of estimating survival probabilities are frequently used in assessment of prognosis. Berkson and Gage (6) have provided an actuarial method for estimating survival curves for patient populations under study. Kaplan and Meier (34) defined a maximum likelihood ("product limit") estimate that gives similar interpretation. These curves are usually known as "survival curves" and permit estimation of percent surviving at any given time after treatment start. In essence, these techniques estimate the distribution of survival times for a selected study group. For pragmatic reasons, clinicians frequently extrapolate from the survival curve to derive predictions of survival for a specific patient.

Gehan (26) has discussed aspects of survival analysis including survivorship and hazard functions. The survivorship function gives the probability that an individual will survive longer than a given time. The hazard function gives the instantaneous probability of death for an individual known to be alive at a given time. It is the death rate per unit time and is analogous to the age-specific mortality rate and mortality intensity function used in demography. Cox (14) has described life table regression methods that permit the simultaneous considerations of the effect of prognostic factors, such as treatment, age, sex, and stage of disease, on the hazard function.

Life table methods are applicable to any cohort exposed to a process that causes attrition over time. Thus the expression "survival" could denote overall survival with "death" as the endpoint, or it could be partitioned into clinical components, such as disease-free (relapse-free) survival and postmetastatic (postrelapse) survival. Other terms, such as "remission," "regression," or "disease control," can be substituted for survival. Here the endpoint would be escape of tumor from control (relapse, recurrence, metastasis).

Appropriate methods of statistical inference can attach estimates of precision and confidence in survival predictions.

Prognostic Factors

In recent years, the survival data for a number of childhood malignancies have been dissected biostatistically (e.g., by stepwise regression analysis) to identify the patient characteristics or groups of characteristics that significantly influence the response (magnitude, duration, rate) or outcome (8).

Recognized as important prognostic determinants in different tumors are such patient characteristics (prognostic factors or parameters) as age, sex, race, site of primary, histopathology, time to metastases, site of metastasis, treatment regimens, certain laboratory findings, and extent of the tumor in the patient. Wherever applicable, the prognostic factors are discussed in the chapters dealing with specific tumors.

The identification of prognostic factors has obvious clinical implications. It permits more valid interpretation of results of clinical studies. Predictions of outcome of treatment can be made with greater certainty. Treatment can be selected and/or modified, depending on the presence or absence of meaningful characteristics. Better insight may be attained regarding the biologic behavior of the disease in the patient under treatment.

Clinical Significance

However phrased, the basic question remains the same: When is a patient cured of cancer? The significance of defining as precisely as possible the magnitude of the risk of failure and the duration of the risk affects patients in at least two ways. First, the patient and the family must plan for future life—both immediate and long range. They need some guidelines as to the best possible estimate of their chances for survival or cure. Second, the clinician must be able to decide, with confidence, when active therapy can be safely discontinued. The intensity of therapy and the nature of the treatment depend on the anticipated duration of such therapy.

Despite increased precision and better documentation of data regarding outcome, the definition of cure remains clinical and statistical. Anecdotal experiences with "late, late" relapses are not uncommon. Disease progression has been noted many years after the time period that had been considered "safe" (73,83). There still remains the possibility that in some cases, therapy (particularly chemotherapy) may simply have altered the pattern of tumor growth (10). Obviously, there is a need to devise means of expressing (and quantitating) the degree of tumor control in biologic terms.

CLINICAL RESEARCH

Objectives

When research is earmarked as "clinical," the objectives of the investigations should have relevance to the disease in the patient and to the patient with the disease. Viewed from this perspective, the major objectives of clinical investigations can be listed as follows:

1. Improvement of rate of cure of cancer.
2. Short of cure, the satisfactory control of disease activity as complete as possible for as long as possible.
3. Refinement of therapy to avoid or to reduce risk of deleterious side effects.
4. Alteration of therapy to improve quality of life.
5. Prospective investigation (recognition, treatment, cure) of acute and late effects of therapy.
6. Early determination of rehabilitation needs of the patient.

7. Determination of biologic characteristics of specific cancers ("natural history").
8. Identification of factors (patient and tumor characteristics) of prognostic significance.
9. Recognition of etiologic factors.
10. Therapeutic approaches to patients with tumor recurrence or metastases.

Methodology

The significant methodologic advances that have occurred in recent years in the techniques of clinical investigation can be categorized under several broad headings:

1. Sophistication in experimental designs and analytical methods.
2. Biostatistical input in protocol development.
3. Standardized and effectively applied quality control.
4. Application of meaningful criteria for assessment of toxicity and treatment results.
5. Multiinstitutional collaborative study of uncommon tumors.

One part of the broad spectrum of basic (laboratory) research goes hand in hand with clinical investigations (41). Pharmacologic and pharmacokinetic studies relate to the application and strategy of chemotherapy and to understanding the effects of treatment and toxicity. Perhaps the most direct application of the laboratory activities concerns drug dosage management.

Recently, de Vita (19) reviewed the evolution of therapeutic research in cancer. Properly devised clinical investigations are laborious and time consuming. The current treatment regimens for cancer nearly always are multidisciplinary. Sufficient numbers of patients are needed to satisfy statistical requirements. For proper interpretation of the study, the data must be accumulated over long periods of years (probably averaging 3 to 5 years for many studies).

The Protocol

The protocol is the manual, a set of guidelines, for clinical research. The questions asked (objectives) are clearly defined. The methodology is spelled out. The data to be recorded are specifically indicated. Statistical estimates and number of patients required are projected. Analytical approaches are described. In all studies, the true significance of a protocol must not be misunderstood. The protocol must be investigation oriented and should not be a detailed, textbook exposition of a given cancer. The protocol is not a "cookbook" recipe for the treatment of cancer; it is used primarily to achieve a given purpose.

Ethical Considerations

"The medical imperatives, ethical quandaries and legal constraints" governing the conduct of research on children constitute important aspects of all clinical investigation (92). The physician and the child and his family face stark realities. Cancer almost always kills if ineffectively or inadequately treated. Even if treated, cure cannot be guaranteed. Treatment itself is associated with varying degrees of morbidity in almost all cases and even with mortality under some circumstances. The late effects of therapy must not be ignored. The risk versus benefit ratio underlies all discussions regarding treatment and investigations. Every therapy decision has a direct bearing on the life or death of the child with cancer (16).

It is important that the physician, family, and patient understand fully the limitations and objectives of treatment, the risks of the treatment (both early and late), and the potentials of available (if any) alternative forms of management.

Consent Form

An absolute requirement of clinical investigation is the informed consent form signed by the patient (or legally responsible person) (29). The signed form indicates that the patient understands the nature of the investigation and that he has willingly agreed to participate. The signed form implicitly and explicitly certifies that the physician has explained in understandable words and that the patient has understood such aspects as the (a) purpose of the investigation, (b) possible benefits of the treatment, (c) manner in which the treatment will be conducted, (d) hazards and discomforts of the procedures, and (e) right of the patient to withdraw consent (without prejudice) at any time and discontinue participation in the investigation.

While clinical experimentation without consent is legally and ethically indefensible, the signed consent form does not necessarily mean that there has been complete communication and understanding. Comprehension of technical terms is difficult. Statistical explanations may have little relevance to the patient himself. Educational, cultural, and religious backgrounds may create problems. The emotional stress as well as socioeconomic pressures can influence significantly the ability (and sometimes willingness) of the patient and family to absorb what is said. These aspects are important, and the clinical investigator must be aware of the nature of the problems that exist (5,16,65,75).

MISCELLANEOUS PROBLEMS

The cancer patient and his family may be unwitting victims of ruthless campaigns to sell ineffective and costly treatments. Of irretrievable consequence is the delay or aborting of effective measures, making treatable situations untreatable and curable conditions incurable. The honest reluctance of physicians to make unwarranted promises of successful outcomes are challenged as inability by merchants of pretension (21).

The poignancy of the continuous threat of death and the highly emotional atmosphere that cancer generates all too frequently invite exploitation by the news media. Premature and fragmentary experimental data are exaggerated completely out of proportion with reality, and extraordinary projections are claimed. Patients with progressive disease do "grasp at straws" and will undergo severe sacrifices to follow up on unfounded recommendations of ill-informed friends.

Various other problems are discussed more appropriately in the chapters that follow. Throughout, the need of meaningful and purposeful communication must be stressed—among the professionals who provide the treatment and between the professionals and the patient (with his family constellation). In particular, the risks of the late effects of therapy are important to the patient.

REFERENCES

1. American Cancer Society (1977): *Cancer Facts and Figures 1978.* American Cancer Society, 31 pp.
2. American Cancer Society (1968): *Manual of Tumor Nomenclature and Coding.* American Cancer Society, 74 pp.
3. Anderson, H. A., Lilis, R., Daum, S. M., Fischbein, A. S., and Selikoff, I. J. (1976): Household-contact asbestos neoplastic risk. *Ann. NY Acad. Sci.,* 271:311–323.
4. Arsenau, J. C., Canellos, G. P., Johnson, R., and de Vita, V. T., Jr. (1977): Risk of new cancers in patients with Hodgkin's disease. *Cancer,* 40:1912–1916.
5. Beecher, H. K. (1966): Consent in clinical experimentation: Myth and reality. *JAMA,* 195:34–35.
6. Berkson, J., and Gage, R. R. (1960): Calculation of survival rates for cancer. *Proc. Staff Meet. Mayo Clin.,* 25:270.
7. Breslow, N. (1978): Perspectives on the statistician's role in cooperative clinical research. *Cancer,* 41:326–332.
8. Breslow, N. E., Palmer, N. F., Hill, L. R., Buring, J., and D'Angio, G. J. (1978): Wilms' tumor: Prognostic factors for patients without metastases at diagnosis. Results of the National Wilms' Tumor Society. *Cancer,* 41:1577–1589.
9. Brody, R. S., Schottenfeld, D., and Reid, A. (1977): Multiple primary cancer risk after therapy for Hodgkin's disease. *Cancer,* 14:1917–1926.
10. Burchenal, J. H. (1974): A giant step forward—if. *N. Engl. J. Med.,* 291:1029–1031.
11. Collins, V. P. (1955): Wilms' tumor: Its behavior and prognosis. *J. La. State Med. Soc.,* 107:474–480.
12. Collins, V. P., Loeffler, R. K., and Tivey, H. (1956): Observations on growth rates of human tumors. *Am. J. Roentgenol. Radiat. Ther. Nucl. Med.,* 76:988–1000.

13. Conard, R. A., Dobyns, R. M., and Sutow, W. W. (1970): Thyroid neoplasia as a late effect of acute exposure to radioiodines in fallout. *JAMA*, 214:316–324.

14. Cox, D. R. (1972): Regression models and life tables. *J. R. Stat. Soc.*, B34:187–202.

15. Cutler, S. J., and Young, J. L., Jr. (editors) (1975): The Third National Cancer Survey: Incidence data. *Natl. Cancer Inst. Monogr.*, 41:1–454.

16. D'Angio, G. J., Clatworthy, H. W., Evans, E. A., Newton, W. A., Jr., and Tefft, M. (1978): Is the risk of morbidity and rare mortality worth the cure? *Cancer*, 41:377–380.

17. D'Angio, G. J., Evans, A. E., Breslow, N., Beckwith, B., Bishop, H., Feigl, P., Goodwin, W., Leape, L. L., Sinks, L. F., Sutow, W., Tefft, M., and Wolff, J. (1976): The treatment of Wilms' tumor. Results of the National Wilms' Tumor Study. *Cancer*, 38:633–646.

18. de Lorimier, A. A., Bragg, K. U., and Linden, G. (1969): Neuroblastoma in childhood. *Am. J. Dis. Child.*, 118:441–450.

19. de Vita, V. T., Jr. (1978): The evolution of therapeutic research in cancer. *N. Engl. J. Med.*, 298:907–910.

20. Draper, G. J., Heaf, M. M., and Wilson, L. M. K. (1977): Occurrence of childhood cancers among sibs and estimation of familial risks. *J. Med. Genet.*, 14:81–90.

21. Faw, C., Ballentine, R., Ballentine, L., and van Eys, J. (1977): Unproved cancer remedies. A survey of use in pediatric outpatients. *JAMA*, 238:1536–1538.

22. Fraumeni, J. F., Jr. (1973): Genetic factors. In: *Cancer Medicine*, edited by J. F. Holland and E. Frei, III, pp. 7–15. Lea & Febiger, Philadelphia.

23. Fraumeni, J. F., Jr. (editor) (1975): *Persons at High Risk of Cancer. An Approach to Cancer Etiology and Control.* 544 pp. Academic, New York.

24. Fraumeni, J. F., Jr. (1977): Clinical patterns of familial cancer. *Prog. Cancer Res. Ther.*, 3:223–233.

25. Frei, E., III, Jaffe, N., Gero, M., Skipper, H., and Watts, H. (1978): Adjuvant chemotherapy of osteogenic sarcoma: Progress and perspectives. *J. Natl. Cancer Inst.*, 60:3–10.

26. Gehan, E. A. (1969): Estimating survival functions from the life table. *J. Chronic Dis.*, 21:629–644.

27. Gehan, E. A., Sutow, W. W., and Uribe-Botero, G. (1978): Osteosarcoma: The M. D. Anderson experience, 1950–1974. In: *Immunotherapy of Cancer: Present Status of Treatment in Man*, edited by W. Terry and D. Windhorst, pp. 271–282. Raven Press, New York.

28. Gross, R. E., Farber, S., and Martin, L. W. (1959): Neuroblastoma sympatheticum. A study and report of 217 cases. *Pediatrics*, 23:1179–1191.

29. Holt, J. (1978): The right of children to informed consent. In: *Research on Children. Medical Imperatives, Ethical Quandaries and Legal Constraints*, edited by J. van Eys, pp. 5–16. University Park Press, Baltimore.

30. Hutchison, G. B. (1976): Late neoplastic changes following medical irradiation. *Cancer*, 37:1102–1107.

31. Jaffe, N. (1976): Neuroblastoma: Review of the literature and an examination of factors contributing to its enigmatic character. *Cancer Treat. Rev.,* 3:61–82.
32. Jereb, B., and Eklund, G. (1973): Factors influencing the cure rate in nephroblastoma. *Acta Radiol. (Ther.),* 12:84–106.
33. Johnson, F. L., Feagler, J. R., Lerner, K. G., Majerus, P. W., Siegel, M., Hartmann, J. R., and Thomas, E. D. (1972): Association of androgenic-anabolic steroid therapy with development of hepatocellular carcinoma. *Lancet,* 2:1273–1276.
34. Kaplan, E. L., and Meier, P. (1958): Nonparametric estimation from incomplete observations. *J. Am. Stat. Assoc.,* 51:457.
35. Kim, J. H., Chu, F. C., Woodard, H. Q., Melamed, M. R., Huvos, A., and Cantin, J. (1978): Radiation-induced soft-tissue and bone sarcoma. *Radiology,* 129:501–508.
36. Knox, W. E., and Pillers, E. M. K. (1958): Time of recurrence or cure of tumours in childhood. *Lancet,* 1:188–191.
37. Knudson, A. G., Jr. (1971): Mutation and cancer: A statistical study of retinoblastoma. *Proc. Natl. Acad. Sci. USA,* 68:820–823.
38. Knudson, A. G., Jr. (1978): Retinoblastoma: A prototypic hereditary neoplasm. *Semin. Oncol.,* 5:57–65.
39. Knudson, A. G., Jr., and Strong, L. C. (1972): Mutation and cancer: A model for Wilms' tumor of the kidney. *J. Natl. Cancer Inst.,* 48:313–324.
40. Knudson, A. G., Jr., and Strong, L. C. (1972): Mutation and cancer: Neuroblastoma and pheochromocytoma. *Am. J. Hum. Genet.,* 24:514.
41. Kornberg, A. (1976): Research, the lifeline of medicine. *N. Engl. J. Med.,* 294:1212–1216.
42. Leck, I. (1977): Congenital malformations and childhood neoplasms. *J. Med. Genet.,* 14:321–326.
43. Li, F. P. (1977): Second malignant tumors after cancer in childhood. *Cancer,* 40:1899–1902.
44. Li, F. P. (1978): Host factors in the development of childhood cancers. *Semin. Oncol.,* 5:17–23.
45. Li, F. P., Fine, W., Jaffe, N., Holmes, G. E., and Holmes, F. F. (1979): Offspring of patients treated for cancer in childhood. *J. Natl. Cancer Inst.,* 62:1193–1197.
46. Li, F. P., and Fraumeni, J. F., Jr. (1975): Familial breast cancer, soft-tissue sarcomas, and other neoplasms. *Ann. Intern. Med.,* 83:833–834.
47. Lynch, P. M., and Lynch, H. T. (1978): Genetic counseling of high-cancer-risk patients: Jurisprudential considerations. *Semin. Oncol.,* 5:107–118.
48. Lynch, H. T., Guirgis, H. A., Lynch, P. M., Lynch, J. F., and Harris, R. E. (1977): Familial cancer syndromes: A survey. *Cancer,* 39:1867–1881.
49. Maurer, H. M., Donaldson, M., Gehan, E. A., Hammond, D., Hays, D. M., Lawrence, W., Jr., Lindberg, R., Newton, W., Ragab, A., Raney, B. V., Ruymann, F., Soule, E. H., Sutow, W. W., and Tefft, M. (1980): The Intergroup Rhabdomyosarcoma Study—update November 1978. *Natl. Cancer Inst. Monogr. (in press).*

50. Maurer, H. M., Moon, T., Donaldson, M., Fernandez, C., Gehan, E. A., Hammond, D., Hays, D. M., Lawrence, W., Jr., Newton, W., Ragab, A., Soule, E. H., Sutow, W. W., and Tefft, M. (1977): The Intergroup Rhabdomyosarcoma Study. A preliminary report. *Cancer,* 40:2015–2026.

51. Maxon, H. R., Thomas, S. R., Saenger, E. L., Buncher, C. R., and Kereiakes, J. G. (1977): Ionizing irradiation and the induction of clinically significant disease in the human thyroid gland. *Am. J. Med.,* 63:967–978.

52. Mays, C. W. (1973): Cancer induction in man from internal radioactivity. *Health Phys.,* 25:585–592.

53. Meadows, A. T., Naiman, J. L., and Valdes-Dapena, M. (1974): Hepatoma associated with androgen therapy for aplastic anemia. *J. Pediatr.,* 84:109–110.

54. Meadows, A. T., D'Angio, G. J., Miké, V., Banfi, A., Harris, C., Jenkin, R. D. T., and Schwartz, A. (1977): Patterns of second malignant neoplasms in children. *Cancer,* 40:1903–1911.

55. Miller, R. W. (1971): Deaths from childhood leukemia and solid tumors among twins and other sibs in the United States. *J. Natl. Cancer Inst.,* 40:203–209.

56. Miller, R. W. (1974): Late radiation effects: Status and needs of epidemiologic research. *Environ. Res.,* 8:221–233.

57. Miller, R. W. (1977): Etiology of childhood cancer. In: *Clinical Pediatric Oncology,* second edition, edited by W. W. Sutow, T. J. Vietti, and D. J. Fernbach, pp. 33–45. C. V. Mosby, St. Louis.

58. Miller, R. W. (1977): Bedside etiology of childhood cancer. *CA,* 27:273–280.

59. Miller, R. W. (1978): Environmental causes of cancer in childhood. *Adv. Pediatr.,* 25:97–119.

60. Miké, V., and Marcove, R. C. (1978): Osteogenic sarcoma under the age of 21: Experience at Memorial Sloan-Kettering Cancer Center. *Prog. Cancer Res. Ther.,* 6:283–292.

61. Modan, B., Baidatz, D., Mart, H., Steinitz, R., and Levin, S. G. (1974): Radiation-induced head and neck tumours. *Lancet,* 1:277–279.

62. Modan, B., Ron, E., and Werner, A. (1977): Thyroid cancer following scalp irradiation. *Radiology,* 123:741–744.

63. Mulvihill, J. J. (1975): Congenital and genetic diseases. In: *Persons at High Risk of Cancer. An Approach to Cancer Etiology and Control,* edited by J. F. Fraumeni, Jr., pp. 3–37. Academic, New York.

64. Mulvihill, J. J., Miller, R. W., and Fraumeni, J. F., Jr. (editors) (1977): *Genetics of Human Cancer,* 519 pp. Raven Press, New York.

65. Muss, H. B., White, D. R., Michieulutte, R., Richards, F., II, Cooper, R., Williams, S., Stuart, J. J., and Spurr, C. L. (1979): Written informed consent in patients with breast cancer. *Cancer,* 43:1549–1556.

66. Nesbit, M., Vietti, T., Burgert, O., Tefft, M., Gehan, E., Perez, C., Razek, A., and Kissane, J. (1978): Intergroup Ewing's Sarcoma Study (IESS): Results of three different treatment regimens. *Proc. AACR ASCO,* 19:81 (Abstr.).

67. O'Brien, P. C., Noller, K. L., Robboy, S. J., Barnes, A. B., Kaufman, R. H., Tilley, B. C., and Townsend, D. E. (1979): Vaginal epithelial changes in young women enrolled in the National Cooperative Diethylstilbestrol Adenosis (DESAD) project. *Obstet. Gynecol.,* 53:300–308.
68. Perez, C. A., Razek, A., Tefft, M., Nesbit, M., Burgert, O., Jr., Kissane, J., Vietti, T., and Gehan, E. A. (1977): Analysis of local tumor control in Ewing's sarcoma. Preliminary results of a cooperative intergroup study. *Cancer,* 40:2864–2873.
69. Platt, B. B., and Linden, G. (1964): Wilms's tumor—A comparison of 2 criteria for survival. *Cancer,* 17:1573–1578.
70. Proceedings of the Conference on Cancer Epidemiology and the Clinician. Boston, Massachusetts, October 23–25, 1975 (1977): *Cancer,* 39:1769–1922.
71. Proceedings of the International Workshop on Multiple Primary Cancers. New York, New York, October 7–8, 1976 (1977): *Cancer,* 40:1785–1985.
72. Refetoff, S., Harrison, J., Karanfilski, B. T., Kaplan, E. L., DeGroot, L. J., and Bekerman, C. (1975): Continuing occurrence of thyroid carcinoma after irradiation to the neck in infancy and childhood. *N. Engl. J. Med.,* 292:171–175.
73. Richards, M. J. S., Joo, P., and Gilbert, E. F. (1976): The rare problem of late recurrence in neuroblastoma. *Cancer,* 38:1847–1852.
74. Robboy, S. J., Kaufman, R. H., Prat, J., Welch, W. R., Gaffey, T., Sculley, R. E., Richart, R., Fenoglio, C. M., Virata, R., and Tilley, B. C. (1979): Pathologic findings in young women enrolled in the National Cooperative Diethylstilbestrol Adenosis (DESAD) Project. *Obstet. Gynecol.,* 53:309–317.
75. Robinson, G., and Merav, A. (1976): Informed consent: Recall by patients tested postoperatively. *Ann. Thorac. Surg.,* 22:209–212.
76. Rosen, G. (1978): Primary Ewing's sarcoma: The multidisciplinary lesion. *Int. J. Radiat. Oncol. Biol. Phys.,* 4:527–532.
77. Rosen, G., Caparros, B., Mosende, C., McCormick, B., Huvos, A. G., and Marcove, R. C. (1978): Curability of Ewing's sarcoma and considerations for future therapeutic trials. *Cancer,* 41:888–899.
78. Rozencweig, M., and Muggia, F. M. (1979): The delta and epsilon errors in the assessment of cancer clinical trials. *Proc. AACR ASCO,* 20:231 (Abstr.).
79. Shimaoka, K., Getaz, E. P., Razack, M. S., Rao, U., Norman, M., Wallace, H. J., Jr., and Shedd, D. P. (1979): Screening program for radiation-associated thyroid carcinoma. *Proc. AACR ASCO,* 20:19 (Abstr.).
80. Silverman, C., and Hoffman, D. A. (1975): Thyroid tumor risk from radiation during childhood. *Prev. Med.,* 4:100–105.
81. Strong, L. C. (1977): Genetic etiology of cancer. *Cancer,* 40:438–444.
82. Strong, L. C. (1977): Genetic considerations in pediatric oncology. In: *Clinical Pediatric Oncology,* second edition, edited by W. W. Sutow, T. J. Vietti, and D. J. Fernbach, pp. 16–32. C. V. Mosby, St. Louis.
83. Sutow, W. W. (1976): Late metastases in osteosarcoma. *Lancet,* 1:856.
84. Sutow, W. W. (1976): Wilms' tumor. *Methods Cancer Res.,* 13:31–65.

85. Sutow, W. W. (1978): Primary adjuvant chemotherapy in osteosarcoma. *Cancer Bull.*, 30:178–181.
86. Sutow, W. W. (1978): Successful control of childhood solid tumors with intensive multimodal treatment. *J. Japan Soc. Cancer Ther.*, 13:44–47.
87. Sutow, W. W. (1979): Wilms' tumor—retrospect and prospect. In: *Proceedings of American Cancer Society National Conference on the Care of the Child with Cancer*, pp. 62–70. Geo. F. Stickley, Philadelphia.
88. Sutow, W. W.: *Unpublished data.*
89. Sutow, W. W., Breslow, N., Palmer, N. F., D'Angio, G. J., and Takashima, J. R. (1979): Prognosis after relapse in children with Wilms' tumor. Results from the first National Wilms' Tumor Study (NWTS-1). *Proc. AACR ASCO*, 20:68 (Abstr.).
90. Sutow, W. W., Herson, J., and Perez, C. (1980): Survival after metastasis in osteosarcoma. *Natl. Cancer Inst. Monogr. (in press).*
91. Thomas, L. B., Popper, H., Berk, P. D., Selikoff, I., and Falk, H. (1975): Vinyl-chloride-induced liver disease. From idiopathic portal hypertension (Banti's syndrome) to angiosarcoma. *N. Engl. J. Med.*, 292:17–22.
92. van Eys, J. (editor) (1978): *Research on Children. Medical Imperatives, Ethical Quandries and Legal Constraints*, 152 pp. University Park Press, Baltimore.
93. Vital Statistics of the United States–1975 (1977): Hyattsville, Md. National Center for Health Statistics. Public Health Service, HEW Vol. II, Part B, Sec. 7, pp. 134–151.
94. Weisburger, E. K. (1977): Bioassay program for carcinogenic hazards of cancer chemotherapeutic agents. *Cancer*, 40:1935–1949.
95. Young, J. L., Jr., Heise, H. W., Silverberg, E., and Myers, M. H. (1978): Cancer incidence, survival and mortality for children under 15 years of age. *Am. Cancer Soc.*, 16 pp.
96. Young, J. L., Jr., and Miller, R. W. (1975): Incidence of malignant tumors in U.S. children. *J. Pediatr.*, 86:254–258.

2

The Child With Cancer

Cancer in children is relatively rare—so much so that Osler's admonition that "unfamiliarity breeds misdiagnosis and poor treatment" (34) seems distressingly appropriate. Thurman (34) has pointed out that among surgeons and pediatricians, there exists an alarmingly low level of awareness of current progress and attitudes toward cancer in children, insufficient to assure best diagnosis and optimal treatment. In the absence of the required expertise, it has been recommended that the child with suspected malignancy be referred to a medical center (34). It is important, therefore, to review the systematic approach to a child who may have cancer (solid tumor).

This systematic approach can be divided arbitrarily into several phases, based on considerations of the defined purposes of the clinical activities conducted during those phases. Briefly, the initial phase is related to the assessment of the patient and the diagnostic intervention. The second phase is concerned with the interpretation of the diagnosis, staging of the disease in the patient, and careful review of the treatment plans. The third phase is treatment, the surgical aspect of which may already have been completed. During the fourth or follow-up phase, the important aspects of the end result of therapy are considered, such as cure of the disease, late effects of therapy, and rehabilitation.

INITIAL PHASE: PRIMARY DIAGNOSTIC EVALUATION

The first phase of management is concerned with the direct evaluation of the patient as a child with potential cancer. A presumptive clinical diagnosis is considered, and the patient is evaluated, first to document all evidence that will strengthen the presumptive diagnosis, and second to seek evidence that may point to a different diagnosis. This phase ends with the establishment of the histopathologic diagnosis from microscopic examination of the tumor tissue.

Since the manifestations of cancer are so protean, the possibility of malignant disease should never be ignored. In children, however, the diagnostic evaluation generally begins after the question of neoplastic disease is raised by development of symptoms or the discovery of clinical abnormalities. In a special category are those children at unusual risk of cancer (12,24). Examples are those who received radiation to the head and neck area including the thyroid (8,14,21,22,38) and those with family history of retinoblastoma or other types of genetically related cancers (24,25). As other potentially carcinogenic circumstances are identified, such as ingestion of diethylstilbestrol (DES) by the mother during pregnancy (15,16) or androgenic anabolic steroids by patients (20), the population at risk will increase.

The latent period required for carcinogenesis may often lead to circumstances where the exposure to the carcinogen, such as DES and vinyl chloride (37), may occur early but the clinical development of cancer may be noted in adulthood. It is obvious that a carefully detailed history, whether positive or negative, may provide etiologic clues regarding the possible nature of the mass in the child.

Present Illness

The history of the present illness should provide the basis for the differential diagnoses to be considered and the diagnostic procedures to be scheduled. The type, duration, and course of symptomatology are important leads to the primary site of the tumor, the extent of the tumor in the patient, and the possible nature and behavior of the tumor. Essentially, the synthesis of information from the history should limit the number of diagnostic possibilities. This allows early thinking about further diagnostic procedures after concomitant assessment of the results of physical examination and of preliminary routine screening tests (such as chest films, blood counts, basic biochemical parameters, and urinalysis).

Physical Examination

One part of the physical examination will be oriented to the tumor problem to eventuate in a presumptive diagnosis (or differential diagnoses) and a concept of the extent of the tumor in the patient. The second purpose of the physical examination is a general pediatric assessment to determine the clinical status of the child, apart from the tumor-related consequences. The independent existence of other medical conditions must not be overlooked. The total therapy currently used in pediatric oncology requires a careful, baseline study of the whole child.

Diagnostic Procedures

The ultimate diagnostic procedure is the surgical excision of the entire tumor or a piece of the tumor for histopathologic examination. Prior to and following such surgery, however, diagnostic studies are essential to guide therapeutic decisions. Primarily, the studies are expected to indicate the nature and extent of the tumor and the site of the primary tumor. Additionally, the studies permit assessment of the effect of the tumor mass on the patient. Because of their therapeutic as well as diagnostic implications, the diagnostic procedures must be purposefully selected in collaboration with members of the management team. Ideally, all potentially helpful studies should be considered, and the maximum amount of information should be obtained. The information then should be collated and digested by the management team so that plans for both diagnosis and therapy can be finalized.

Establish Nature of the Tumor

In almost every case, the surgical biopsy (or the surgical tumor specimen) provides the material for study by the pathologist.

Before, during, and after the diagnosis has been made, however, there must be a purposeful planning of the approach to the patient. A presumptive working diagnosis (or limited differential diagnosis) must be established to guide the choice and sequence of diagnostic procedures to be utilized. Decision must be made regarding the site and extent of surgery for diagnostic purposes (e.g., incisional or excisional biopsy). Even the placement of the surgical scar from the biopsy must be determined with forethought of the diagnostic possibilities. A scar resulting from a hastily done biopsy, for example, may impair the proper administration of subsequent radiation therapy or require additional surgical procedures.

Select Appropriate Diagnostic Procedures

Biochemical markers, if present, may be helpful both in indicating the probable nature of the tumor before histologic studies and in monitoring disease activity during and after therapy.

Radiologic studies are essential in determining the extent of the disease. Recent developments in radionuclide imaging and ultrasonography can provide sophisticated information on tumor site and extent and even characterization of mass lesions (13,23). The diagnostic radiologist may be invaluable in performing percutaneous puncture of organs and organ lesions under fluoroscopic and ultrasound guidance for diagnostic purposes. Computed tomography adds still another important dimension to precise documentation of the location, extent, and even nature of mass lesions (1).

Determine Extent of the Tumor

It is essential to determine as accurately as possible the extent of the tumor in the patient. The primary site must be established. The degree and anatomic locations of extension and metastases must be documented. The specifics of the tumor should be accurately recorded in the patient's chart (a) as completely as possible, (b) objectively, and (c) in quantitative terms.

The presumptive diagnosis must be kept in mind constantly

since the biopsy procedure itself, which may be complete extirpation of the tumor, will depend on whether the tumor is localized, locally extensive, or disseminated. Subsequent staging of the disease in the patient, as well as the treatment program, will be based on the knowledge of the amount and location of the tumor.

Assess Effect of Tumor on Patient

A malignant solid tumor consists of a mass that, without response to therapy, will display its inherent behavior, increasing inexorably in size and developing distant metastases. By pressure on body structures, by replacement, and by destruction of normal tissues, the growing tumor produces anatomic and functional distortions, disabilities, and defects. Depending on the location, extent, and severity, the deleterious effects of the tumor on the patient will require assessment and therapy. More important, the presence and magnitude of the tumor effects may influence the intensity and sequence of the treatment modalities.

Evaluate Capacity to Undergo Therapy

By the very nature of the problem to which it is directed, successful cancer therapy is usually intensive and prolonged. It is necessary to assess the potential capacity of the patient to absorb satisfactorily the physical and physiologic stress of the treatment. The planning of the treatment program must include contingency provisions, should significant deficiencies exist or develop in the patient. Meaningful corrective efforts must be made to restore the patient to the best possible condition for the therapy and to maintain the patient in a clinically acceptable status.

INITIAL PHASE: SECONDARY DIAGNOSTIC EVALUATION

Socioeconomic Evaluation

Cancer treatment is costly in terms of money, time, and disruption of normal life activities; the necessary patient care drains rapidly and steadily all the family resources. It is important that some assessment be made of how the family is prepared to meet these demands of travel, prolonged hospitalization, frequent outpatient visits, absence from school, and stress of rehabilitation programs.

Such assessments must be made early and repeated regularly during the treatment program. Inevitably, these practical considerations may affect the capacity of the family despite their desires and willingness to adhere to the requirements of maximum care. In these activities, the physican requires especially the collaboration of the nurse, public health nurse, and social worker.

Psychosocial Impact

The existence of an imminent catastrophic threat, actual or potential, produces severe strains within the family constellation and its relationship to the community and society. The anticipation and management of these emotional reactions constitute an important area that requires independent, specialized, and expert approach, again in a multidisciplinary manner (including the clinicians, mental health specialists, nursing personnel, social workers, and clergy, among others).

The physician must be alert to the possible existence of some complicating problems that may impact directly on the planned treatment programs. For example, the medical, legal, and ethical considerations in patients of the Jehovah's Witness faith, who may have urgent indications for transfusions of blood products, constitute a challenge (11). Unless satisfactorily resolved, the religious constraints may necessitate relaxation of the required intensity of the entire treatment program in efforts to avoid myelosuppression from drugs.

Ingrained cultural teachings occasionally create obstacles to the orderly sequence of planned therapy and generate possible hazards for the child. The surreptitious administration of home remedies may substitute for or be added to the prescribed medications. Serious consequences usually result from the delay or omission of effective measures.

Personal prejudices on the part of the patients are frequently strengthened by the honest admission of the physician that he cannot guarantee results or make accurate predictions regarding outcome. Complications and unsatisfactory tumor control may make the parents extremely susceptible to unscrupulous advertisements and to urgings of well-meaning but uninformed relatives and friends. Pressure, often heavy, is exerted to discontinue conventional treatment and to accept unestablished and professionally unaccepted forms of management. Families may profess intense adherence to food fads or occasionally to some unusual nutritionally oriented beliefs.

The potential existence of personal convictions that are likely to interfere with planned therapy should be sought. Frank and repeated discussions with the parents are helpful, and free communication must be maintained. It is particularly important that willful therapeutic digressions on the part of the parents do not result in the omission of key procedures or drugs in the planned treatment program.

Past History and Family History

Past medical illnesses may relate importantly to some aspects of therapy. For example, a history of cardiopathy, renal disease, or pulmonary problems would engender cautionary alerts in the consideration of some chemotherapeutic agents or of general anesthesia.

Details of the past history and family history may provide possible clues to the etiology of the tumor. This information may be particularly pertinent if risk to other family members needs to be projected. Such background data may be helpful in genetic counseling for the survivor and family under some circumstances. The eventual scientific value of well-documented data in all patients is obvious. (This aspect is mentioned earlier in this chapter.)

SECOND PHASE: POSTDIAGNOSIS/PRETREATMENT

In this chapter, the period between the determination of diagnosis and onset of postsurgical therapy has been arbitrarily designated the second phase of evaluation. This relatively short interval is utilized to reconfirm the apparent clinical stage of the disease, to anticipate the biologic behavior of the tumor, to carefully review the plan of therapy, and to ascertain the understanding of the disease and the further treatment details by the child and the parents.

Staging

In most solid tumors, the clinical stage is an important determinant of prognosis or outcome, measured as duration of disease control, degree of tumor control, and curability. In such cancers as Wilms' tumor (9,10) and rhabdomyosarcoma (19), clinical staging techniques have already been field tested and validated. The criteria include both extent of the anatomic involvement of the tumor (localized, regional, metastatic) and the degree of residual tumor after primary surgery (no residuum, microscopic residuum, gross residual tumor, disseminated tumor). The details of these staging techniques are further described in the chapters on the specific tumors.

Staging of pediatric solid tumors now has a more complex and significant implication than the mere description of anatomic distribution of neoplastic tissue. As exemplified in Wilms' tumor, the concept of staging includes not only an assessment of the degree to which surgical extirpation of the tumor load was possible (9,17) but also the histopathologic estimate of the degree of malignancy of the tumor (2). Once precision and reliability are established, the staging results are used to determine both treatment planning and prediction of prognosis.

Prediction of Biologic Behavior

For every solid tumor, significant prognostic factors must be utilized in the design of the therapeutic approach (4). While the histopathologic "degree of malignancy" has been discussed over the years for many tumors, the difficulties in clearly identifying the patterns in actual situations had precluded their clinical usefulness. Ganglioneuroblastoma, for example, was and is considered to demonstrate less aggressive activity than a straightforward neuroblastoma (3,18). The desmoid tumors are considered by some to be at the benign end of a spectrum of fibrosarcomas (7). In Wilms' tumor, the relationship of histopathology to prognosis was clearly demonstrated, and several types of prognostically unfavorable histologic patterns were identified (2). The separation of the prognostically unfavorable histologic tumors will permit selective intensification of treatment programs for those patients. Another facet to the more refined approach to histopathologic characterization is the possibility that metastatic behavior also may be predictable to some degree. Data from studies of Wilms' tumor, for example, suggest that bone metastases occur almost exclusively with the "clear cell" anaplasia rhabdoid type (2).

Information regarding other determinants of behavior and prognosis exists. For example, in rhabdomyosarcoma, the site of the primary tumor has certain therapeutic and biologic implications. Tumors arising in the extremities appear to be less well controlled than those arising in other sites, irrespective of the histologic type and therapy (19,26). Tumors arising in the head and neck areas, specifically in the parameningeal sites, carry a significant potentiality (35%, 20/57) of spreading to the central nervous system area (33). Such progression means almost certain death (33).

For many years, it has been noted that age was correlated with survival, the younger children having better survival rates than older children for such tumors as Wilms' tumor (27) and neuroblastoma (5,27,28). Therefore, the age factor may have to be considered in the development, selection, and application of the intensive therapeutic regimens.

Even after primary treatment fails and metastases occur, successful treatment has achieved "retrieval" and long-term survival in patients with such cancers as Wilms' tumor (29) and osteosarcoma (30). Analyses of prognostic factors indicate in both tumors that the time interval between diagnosis and metastases is directly correlated with postmetastatic survival.

Planning of Therapy

The integration of the many considerations into a planned therapeutic program is discussed above and also in the chapter on multimodal therapy. In essence, the objectives of the treatment and the impact of the various factors determine the final approach. The exact nature of the therapy plan will depend on the specific cancer under consideration and is discussed more appropriately in chapters dealing with individual tumors.

Consent (Assent) Form

This important form, signed by the patient and by the parents, indicates first that discussions have been held. Second, the patient and the parents certify that they understand the clinical problems generated by the tumor, the treatment plans for the tumor, and the nature of the treatment. Furthermore, the form indicates that the uncertainties of the results and the possible deleterious effects (acute, chronic, and late) of therapy have been explained. The form finally documents that the patient and the parents will accept the treatment. The signature affirms that alternative forms of treatment (to the degree applicable to the clinical situation present) have been discussed and that the patient may terminate, without prejudice, the treatment program at any time.

Treatment programs for childhood solid tumors are becoming increasingly complex. Certain phases or the entire program may be "investigative" in approach (31). The patient and/or responsible family members must understand the risks and uncertainties of all such aspects (35). Therapeutic research in childhood cancer includes two overriding medical considerations. First, there is the need to continually improve therapeutic effectiveness for any specific cancer until survival can be achieved for all children with that cancer. Second, there is the concomitant imperative to refine therapy whenever possible, so that maximum treatment result can be achieved with minimum morbidity (acute or late) to the patient.

THIRD PHASE: TREATMENT

The conceptual aspects of therapy for childhood cancer are outlined in the chapter on multimodal therapy. The practical details of therapeutic programs are discussed in the sections on specific tumors. Temporally, the entire treatment program can be considered as a sequence of events with alternate courses to follow, depending on the failure or success of the therapeutic efforts at any given point.

The central objective of primary treatment is the eradication of all tumor tissue (cure). Cure may be considered to have occurred early in some situations, such as in stage I Wilms' tumor where nephrectomy and adjuvant chemotherapy are curative. In other cases, the control of tumor may be temporary (remission/ regression) with eventual regrowth of tumor after variable periods of time. Relapse from therapy may occur as local recurrence or distant metastases, or both. Even after relapse or metastases (in some cases more than once), further curative therapy can be successful (29,30).

When cure cannot be achieved, meaningful palliation is attempted. Here the purpose is to maintain the maximum degree of tumor control for as long as possible.

In unsuccessful cases, the control of tumor eventually fails, and the patient will be unresponsive to all forms of available treatment. During this so-called "terminal" period of illness, maximum degree of symptomatic palliation is attempted with minimum discomfort to the patient.

FOURTH PHASE: FOLLOW-UP PROGRAM

During the fourth phase, the result of therapy on the tumor is monitored, and the untoward effects of therapy on the patient are assessed. Also, the defects caused by the tumor and by treatment of the tumor are identified, and corrective procedures are instituted. It is the aim to maintain the quality of life for the survivor at the most optimal level possible.

Tumor-Oriented Follow-Up

During this phase, the result of antitumor therapy is periodically evaluated to determine the degree and quality of tumor control. Thus the follow-up diagnostic studies are intended to detect any local recurrence of the tumor and to demonstrate any evidence of metastatic disease. When the initial therapy results in apparently complete tumor eradication, the risk of disease relapse subsequently decreases with increasing duration of time from therapy. In such situations, the frequency of examinations is progressively lessened, from monthly examinations during the first year to bimonthly check-ups during the second year, to semi-annual studies during the third year. Thereafter, annual examinations usually suffice. If there had been metastatic disease or incomplete tumor eradication, the patient is followed more closely and at more frequent intervals for a longer period.

It has been postulated that the so-called "period of risk" beyond which relapse is extremely uncommon was considered to be about 2 years for such tumors as neuroblastoma, Wilms' tumor, and rhabdomyosarcoma. More recently, the possibility has been suggested that intensive chemotherapy in some cases may simply delay the appearance of tumor relapse (6). Metastases or local tumor relapses occurring many years later have been noted (32).

Effect of Therapy on the Patient

During the follow-up phase, the patients undergo careful and systematic examinations to detect the deleterious late effects of therapy. Evaluations of the pattern of growth and development and measures of physiologic functions are conducted. Various aspects of this phase of the follow-up program are discussed in the chapter, "Cost of Survival."

Rehabilitation Program

Rehabilitation, an important aspect of pediatric oncology, is one of the least well-developed programs even in cancer centers. Often as the result of injury caused by the presence of tumor mass but more often as the result of the necessary treatment, varying degrees of physiologic and physical disabilities remain. They need carefully planned rehabilitative treatment.

Of greater benefit to the patient is the anticipation of the problems and the institution of programs with prophylactic intent (36).

REFERENCES

1. Alfidi, R. J. (editor) (1977): Symposium on computed body tomography. *Radiol. Clin. North Am.,* 15:295–469.
2. Beckwith, J. B., and Palmer, N. F. (1978): Histopathology and prognosis of Wilms' tumor. *Cancer,* 41:1937–1948.
3. Beckwith, J. B., and Perrin, E. V. (1963): In situ neuroblastomas: A contribution to the natural history of neural crest tumors. *Am. J. Pathol.,* 43:1089–1104.
4. Breslow, N. E., Palmer, N. F., Hill, L. R., Buring, J., and D'Angio, G. J. (1978): Wilms' tumor: Prognostic factors for patients without metastases at diagnosis. Results of the National Wilms' Tumor Study. *Cancer,* 41:1577–1589.
5. Breslow, N., and McCann, B. (1971): Statistical estimation of prognosis for children with neuroblastoma. *Cancer Res.,* 31:2098–2103.
6. Burchenal, J. H. (1974): A giant step forward—if. (Editorial.) *N. Engl. J. Med.,* 291:1029–1031.
7. Butler, J. J. (1965): Fibrous tissue tumors: Nodular fasciitis, dermatofibrosarcoma, protuberans, and fibrosarcoma, Grade 1, desmoid type. In: *Tumors of Bone and Soft Tissue,* pp. 397–413. Year Book, Chicago.
8. Conard, R. A., Dobyns, B. M., and Sutow, W. W. (1970): Thyroid neoplasia as a late effect of acute exposure to radioiodines in fallout. *JAMA,* 214:316–324.
9. D'Angio, G. J., Beckwith, J. B., Bishop, H. C., Breslow, N., Evans, A. E., Goodwin, W. E., King, L. R., Pickett, L. K., Sinks, L. F., Sutow,

W. W., and Wolff, J. A. (1973): The National Wilms' Tumor Study: A progress report. In: *Seventh National Cancer Conference Proceedings,* pp. 627–636. Lippincott, Philadelphia.

10. D'Angio, G. J., Evans, A. E., Breslow, N., Beckwith, B., Bishop, H., Feigl, P., Goodwin, W., Leake, L. L., Sinks, L. F., Sutow, W., Tefft, M., and Wolff, J. (1976): The treatment of Wilms' tumor. Results of the National Wilms' Tumor Study. *Cancer,* 38:633–646.

11. Frankel, L. S., Damme, C. J., and van Eys, J. (1977): Childhood cancer and the Jehovah's Witness faith. *Pediatrics,* 60:916–921.

12. Fraumeni, J. F., Jr. (editor) (1975): *Persons at High Risk of Cancer: An Approach to Cancer Etiology and Control.* Academic, New York.

13. Green, B., and Bree, R. L. (1977): Newer techniques in pediatric oncologic radiology. In: *Clinical Pediatric Oncology,* second edition, edited by W. W. Sutow, T. J. Vietti, and D. J. Fernbach, pp. 66–101. C. V. Mosby, St. Louis.

14. Hempelmann, L. H., Hall, W. J., Phillips, M., Cooper, R. A., and Ames, W. R. (1975): Neoplasms in persons treated with x-rays in infancy: Fourth survey in 20 years. *J. Natl. Cancer Inst.,* 55:519–530.

15. Herbst, A. L., Poskanzer, D. C., Robboy, S. J., Friedlander, L., and Scully, R. E. (1975): Prenatal exposure to stilbestrol. A prospective comparison of exposed female offspring with unexposed controls. *N. Engl. J. Med.,* 292:334–339.

16. Herbst, A. L., Cole, P., Colton, T., Robboy, S. J., and Scully, R. E. (1977): Age-incidence and risk of diethylstilbestrol-related clear cell adenocarcinoma of the vagina and cervix. *Am. J. Obstet. Gynecol.,* 128:43–50.

17. Leape, L., Breslow, N., and Bishop, H. C. (1978): The surgical treatment of Wilms' tumor: Results of the National Wilms' Tumor Study. *Ann. Surg.,* 187:351–356.

18. Mäkinen, J. (1972): Microscopic patterns as a guide to prognosis of neuroblastoma in childhood. *Cancer,* 29:1637–1646.

19. Maurer, H. M., Moon, T., Donaldson, M., Fernandez, C., Gehan, E. A., Hammond, D., Hays, D. M., Lawrence, W., Jr., Newton, W., Ragab, A., Raney, B., Soule, E. H., Sutow, W. W., and Tefft, M. (1977): The Intergroup Rhabdomyosarcoma Study: A preliminary report. *Cancer,* 40:2015–2026.

20. Meadows, A. T., Naiman, J. L., and Valdes-Dapena, M. (1974): Hepatoma associated with androgen therapy for aplastic anemia. *J. Pediatr.,* 84(1):109–110.

21. Modan, B., Mart, H., Baidatz, D., Steinitz, R., and Levin, S. G. (1974): Radiation-induced head and neck tumours. *Lancet,* 1:277–278.

22. Refetoff, S., Harrison, J., Karanfilski, B. T., Kaplan, E. L., DeGroot, L. J., and Bekerman, C. (1975): Continuing occurrence of thyroid carcinoma after irradiation to the neck in infancy and childhood. *N. Engl. J. Med.,* 292:171–175.

23. Siegel, B. A., and McIlmoyle, G. (1977): Nuclear imaging in pediatric oncology. In: *Clinical Pediatric Oncology,* second edition, edited by W. W. Sutow, T. J. Vietti, and D. J. Ferbach, pp. 102–127. C. V. Mosby, St. Louis.

24. Strong, L. C. (1977): Genetic considerations in pediatric oncology. In: *Clinical Pediatric Oncology,* second edition, edited by W. W. Sutow, T. J. Vietti, and D. J. Fernbach, pp. 16–32. C. V. Mosby, St. Louis.
25. Strong, L. C. (1977): Genetic etiology of cancer. *Cancer,* 40:438–444.
26. Sutow, W. W., Sullivan, M. P., Ried, H. L., Taylor, H. G., and Griffith, K. M. (1970): Prognosis in childhood rhabdomyosarcoma. *Cancer,* 25:1384–1390.
27. Sutow, W. W., Gehan, E. A., Heyn, R. M., Kung, F. H., Miller, R. W., Murphy, M. L., and Traggis, D. G. (1970): Comparison of survival curves, 1956 versus 1962, in children with Wilms' tumor and neuroblastoma. *Pediatrics,* 45:800–811.
28. Sutow, W. W. (1958): Prognosis in neuroblastoma of childhood. *Am. J. Dis. Child.,* 96:299–305.
29. Sutow, W. W., Breslow, N., Palmer, N. F., D'Angio, G. J., and Takashima, J. R. (1979): Prognosis after relapse in children with Wilms' tumor. Results from the First National Wilms' Tumor Study (NWTS-1). *Proc. AACR ASCO,* 19:68 (Abstr.).
30. Sutow, W. W., Herson, J., and Perez, C. (1980): Survival after metastasis in osteosarcoma. *Natl. Cancer Inst. Monogr. (in press).*
31. Sutow, W. W. (1978): Therapeutic research as a necessary mode of management. In: *Research on Children—Medical Imperatives, Ethical Considerations, Legal Constraints,* edited by J. van Eys, pp. 21–26. University Park Press, Baltimore.
32. Sutow, W. W. (1976): Late metastases in osteosarcoma. *Lancet,* 1:856.
33. Tefft, M., Fernandez, C., Donaldson, M., Newton, W., and Moon, T. (1978): Incidence of meningeal involvement by rhabdomyosarcoma of the head and neck in children. A report of the Intergroup Rhabdomyosarcoma Study (IRS). *Cancer,* 42:253–258.
34. Thurman, W. G. (1976): General aspects of the diagnosis of malignancy in children. In: *Trends in Childhood Cancer,* edited by M. H. Donaldson and H. G. Seydel, pp. 1–5. Wiley, New York.
35. van Eys, J. (editor) (1978): *Research on Children—Medical Imperatives, Ethical Quandaries, and Legal Constraints.* University Park Press, Baltimore.
36. Villanueva, R., and Ajmani, C. P. (1977): Principles of total care—rehabilitation. In: *Clinical Pediatric Oncology,* second edition, edited by W. W. Sutow, T. J. Vietti, and D. J. Fernbach, pp. 276–290. C. V. Mosby, St. Louis.
37. Waxweiler, R. J., Stringer, W., Wagoner, J. K., Jones, J., Falk, H., and Carter, C. (1976): Neoplastic risk among workers exposed to vinyl chloride. *Ann. NY Acad. Sci.,* 271:40–48.
38. Wood, J. W., Tamagaki, H., Neriishi, S., Sato, T., Sheldon, W. F., Archer, P. G., Hamilton, H. B., and Johnson, K. G. (1969): Thyroid carcinoma in atomic bomb survivors, Hiroshima and Nagasaki. *Am. J. Epidemiol.,* 89:4–14.

3

Multimodal Therapy

DEFINITION

Multimodal therapy is the preplanned, coordinated, purposeful use of more than one mode of treatment either concurrently or sequentially to achieve maximum results in the treatment of cancer (4,5,8). Synonyms are multidisciplinary therapy, integrated therapy, and total care. The components of such therapy include all known modes of treatment that have individually demonstrated antitumor capabilities. Currently, the major approaches are surgery, radiotherapy, chemotherapy, and still to a limited extent, immunotherapy.

By implication, the outcome of such therapy should be at least the summation of the results that can be achieved by each modality applied singly. The outcome of therapy can be measured in two ways: (a) improvement of rate and/or duration of disease control, and (b) modification of clinical status by one modality to achieve more effective application of another modality, either by permitting a more intensive program or by decreasing the intensity needed, thus reducing the risk of undesirable side effects.

THE MULTIDISCIPLINARY MANAGEMENT TEAM

The team should include every specialist who can contribute to an optimal end result. Each should meet two requirements: expertise and experience. Depending on the clinical situation, the major responsibilities may shift from one specialist or combination of specialists to another. Burchenal (1) more recently emphasized another essential requirement for an effective working relationship by indicating that the "pride of discipline must be put aside."

The core of the management team on whom the major decision-making responsibilities will fall are the (a) pediatric oncologist/chemotherapist, (b) surgical specialist, (c) pathologist, and (d) diagnostic radiologist.

Equally as important are the back-up personnel who participate actively during special phases of the management program. Such members include the (a) nursing personnel, (b) physiatrist, (c) psychosocial support personnel, (d) geneticist, (e) immunologist, and (f) other basic scientists, such as the pharmacologist.

For the proper functioning of the management team, certain guidelines must be observed:

1. Collaboration must be concurrent (simultaneous) and integrated. Team members must agree on the general plan and must be aware of the timing and purpose of their specific therapeutic contribution. The key activities must be coordinated in the context of the overall objective.
2. Continuous and purposeful communication among the team members is critical.
3. Adequate laboratory back-up should be immediately available for proper monitoring of the current intensive and complex treatment program.
4. Facilities for adequate physiologic support are essential to treat acute effects of therapy.
5. Facilities and personnel must be able to provide adequate and up-to-date clinical care for the child.

OBJECTIVES OF MULTIDISCIPLINARY THERAPY

To provide a perspective, the major objectives of the treatment programs can be listed as follows:

1. *Decrease failure rate.* By so doing, the maximum cure rate (or duration of control) can be achieved.
2. *Refine treatment techniques.* Techniques must be refined to provide optimum results with the least degree of treatment needed. This will minimize toxicity, reduce disability, and

decrease the frequency and intensity of deleterious late effects. Examples are the elimination of radical surgery (avoidance of exenteration in pelvic rhabdomyosarcoma and limb salvage procedures in osteosarcoma) and decrease (or even elimination) in dose/volume of tissues irradiated (in certain clinical groups of Wilms' tumor and rhabdomyosarcoma).

3. *Salvage metastatic cases.* Failures from initial definitive therapy can be salvaged in many instances by prompt, purposeful retreatment.

4. *Define biologic behavior of tumor.* Knowledge of the biologic behavior of the tumor under treatment is an important determinant of the nature, intensity, and sequence of treatments.

5. *Recognize prognostic factors.* Factors that correlate with eventual outcome (such as site of primary tumor, extent of disease, histopathologic pattern, and age) must be identified. Their use as potential determinants of therapy (type and intensity) must be continuously assessed. High risk situations (e.g., risk of central nervous system complications with rhabdomyosarcoma of the head and neck) must be recognized and plans for prophylactic therapy formulated.

6. *Provide adequate follow-up.* Systematic follow-up assessments of the patient are necessary to determine the continued control of tumor. Relapses or metastases should be detected as promptly as possible. Rehabilitation programs must be instituted, and the patient's general condition must be monitored. Genetic counseling may be provided as required.

PRACTICAL OBJECTIVES OF THERAPY

The general objectives of treatment outlined above can be more specifically defined at the practical level as follows: (a) eradicate primary lesion, (b) eradicate micrometastases, (c) eradicate macrometastases, (d) decrease tumor burden, (e) decelerate rate of tumor growth, (f) maintain tumor control as completely and as long as possible, and (g) maximize meaningful palliation when tumor control fails.

STRATEGY OF THERAPY

Looking primarily at cancer therapy in the adult today, Carter and Soper (2) pointed to "the conflict between modality-oriented development and disease-oriented strategy." The approach to almost all pediatric solid tumors is geared to multidisciplinary management. There is prospective planning of diagnostic and therapeutic procedures. Regardless of the degree of difficulty inherent in the clinical problem, a positive attitude is maintained. A planned, persistent, all-out effort is mounted.

Conceptually, the multimodal approach utilizes application of a given modality (a) to modify the extent, intensity, and/or duration of another modality, (b) to increase the effectiveness of another modality, and (c) to decrease the "toxicity" of another modality.

The basic principles outlined for multidrug chemotherapy can be appropriately applied to multimodal treatment programs:

1. Each modality must be independently effective (although varying in degree of effectiveness) against the tumor.
2. Each modality must be capable of eradicating tumor by a different mechanism (e.g., local target-limited action of surgery and irradiation versus systemic action of chemotherapy).
3. Each modality can be utilized at full therapeutic intensity.
4. The major side effects of therapy are different, so that problems of overlapping "toxicity" can be minimized.
5. It must be assumed that the cure rate is less than 100% without the addition of a given modality. One exception here would be the substitution of one modality for another (for tactical reasons). Another exception would be the potential of one modality to permit "refinement" of the intensity of treatment by another modality (6). An example is the

preoperative use of vincristine in Wilms' tumor to facilitate surgery (7).

LIMITING FACTORS

Although there has been significant improvement in the therapeutic effectiveness of a number of treatment approaches, factors may exist in specific patients that limit the appropriate application of the treatment. These factors include:

1. *Mass (size/volume of tumor).* The tumor may be too large for the application of one or more types of therapy.
2. *Site/extent of tumor.* In many circumstances, the location of the tumor will preclude extirpation of the mass by surgery or the sterilization of the tumor by irradiation. Similarly, tumor in sanctuary sites may be protected from systemically administered chemotherapy.
3. *Sensitivity of tumor.* Tumors vary in their susceptibility to the antitumor effects of radiation and drugs. Tumors resistant to these two modes of therapy will survive and continue to progress. Particularly in chemotherapy, the development of resistance is a frequent and frustrating catastrophe that must be recognized early to permit modification of treatment.
4. *Tolerance of treatment.* For optimum effect, the patient must tolerate the effective therapeutic intensity of each of the modalities utilized. Satisfactory tolerance will depend partly on the nature and intensity of the required treatment itself and partly on the clinical status of the patient (extent of tumor, residual effects of prior treatment, physiologic impact of tumor on the patient).

TERMINAL CARE

Despite current advances in treatment, the cancer is not always controlled. The management of a dying child with progressively

growing and spreading tumor taxes to the utmost the skill, pa-
tience, and compassion of the oncologist and his/her colleagues.
The resilience and tolerance of the family members sometimes
disintegrate into a frantic cacophony of accusations and demands
directed at the patient care team, particularly the nurses.

Donaldson (3) has indicated the difficult problems associated
with this phase of patient care. He has emphasized the importance
of a "stable corps" of experienced and dedicated nurses and social
workers in the handling of the terminally ill child or adolescent
and the family. Donaldson (3) further mentions the aspect of
professional responsibility that is frequently overlooked, "the time
after death." Restabilization and reorientation of sense of values
and normalization of family activities after the patients' deaths
are goals toward which the health care team can provide support
and assistance even before the death of the child.

PROJECTIONS

The relative interactions among the three major treatment
modalities (surgery, chemotherapy, and radiotherapy) along with

TABLE 1. *Relative effectiveness of treatment modality in specific solid tumors of childhood*

Tumor	Surgery	Radio-therapy	Chemo-therapy	Immuno-therapy
Osteosarcoma	A	C	B	C
Ewing's sarcoma	B	A	B	D
Wilms' tumor	A	A	A	D
Neuroblastoma	A	A	A	C
Rhabdomyosarcoma	A	A	A	C
Retinoblastoma	A	A	C	D
Brain tumor	A	A	C	D

[a] A, prime therapeutic modality; B, important adjuvant modality; C, investigate approach with some provocative results; D, no definite therapeutic results reported.

immunotherapy with respect to the more commonly encountered childhood solid tumors are indicated in Table 1. While the empiric application of these modalities has resulted in considerable gains, even greater effectiveness can be anticipated as increased knowledge about the behavior of cancer will permit more rational, scientific utilization of the modalities in the patient.

REFERENCES

1. Burchenal, J. H. (1976): Adjuvant therapy—theory, practice, and potential. *Cancer,* 37:46–57.
2. Carter, S. K., and Soper, W. T. (1974): Integration of chemotherapy into combined modality treatment of solid tumors. 1. The overall strategy. *Cancer Treat. Rev.,* 1:1–13.
3. Donaldson, M. H. (1976): The multidisciplinary team approach to the care of children with cancer. In: *Trends in Childhood Cancer,* edited by M. Donaldson and H. G. Seydel, pp. 7–13. Wiley, New York.
4. Farber, S. (1966): Chemotherapy in the treatment of leukemia and Wilms' tumor. *JAMA,* 198:826–836.
5. Farber, S. (1969): The control of cancer in children. In: *Neoplasia in Childhood.* pp. 321–327. Year Book, Chicago.
6. Ortega, J. A., Rivard, G. E., Isaacs, H., Hittle, R. E., Hays, D. M., Pike, M. C., and Karon, M. R. (1975): The influence of chemotherapy on the prognosis of rhabdomyosarcoma. *Med. Pediatr. Oncol.,* 1:227–234.
7. Sullivan, M. P., Sutow, W. W., Cangir, A., and Taylor, G. (1967): Vincristine sulfate in management of Wilms' tumor. Replacement of preoperative irradiation by chemotherapy. *JAMA,* 202:381–384.
8. Sutow, W. W. (1978): Successful control of childhood solid tumors with intensive multimodal treatment. *J. Japan Soc. Cancer Ther.,* 13:44–47.

4

Chemotherapy

Chemotherapy constitutes a major component of multimodal (multidisciplinary) treatment of childhood cancer for both hematolymphatic malignancies and solid tumors (81,83). The rationale, concepts, and practice of chemotherapy have become increasingly complex. The reader is referred to clinical treatises (1,7,19,38, 53,76) and other publications for information on fundamental aspects of the subject, such as the chemistry and biochemistry of the agents (2,44), the pharmacology and pharmacokinetics of the drugs in the human body (12,16,17,57,60), and the basic mechanisms of action and cell cycle specificity (44,51,63,89,90). In this clinically oriented summation of chemotherapy of childhood solid tumors, the relative effectiveness of various drugs and drug combinations is tabulated. The clinical situations in which the drugs have been useful are indicated. The dose schedules and major toxicities are also summarized to provide a concise working reference. This chapter also examines combination drug regimens that have demonstrated significant clinical activity against specific tumor types.

With respect to the chemotherapy of solid tumors, it is emphasized that drugs constitute just one facet of the multimodal approach. The reader is asked to review the chapter on any individual tumor for an assessment of the interrelationship among the treatment modalities.

Among the problems that have been identified but have not been satisfactorily resolved are the acquisition of resistance by the tumor against the drug (41) and the need for means for predicting drug sensitivity (40,41).

The historic development of clinical cancer chemotherapy was recently reviewed by Burchenal (5). A pioneer investigator in the field, Burchenal himself has contributed to many of the major investigative activities.

Utilizing the term "selective toxicity" to indicate specific anticancer effect, Zubrod (92) has listed tumor heterogeneity, cumbersome methodology, and slow pace of clinical studies among the problems in cancer chemotherapy. He has assessed the probability of certain research activities contributing to reduction in cancer mortality in 10 years. He gives research in enhancing selective drug action by tumor manipulation a high probability of success. Research on earlier diagnosis, better adjuvant regimens, and manipulation of drugs are considered to have moderate probability of producing improved results. Manipulation of host, such as better supportive care and rescue techniques, may be helpful. The empiric search for better drugs and better combinations, in Zubrod's opinion, may have reached a plateau (92). The potential benefits of such approaches are now being counterbalanced by the complexities of the regimens and by the increasing array of acute and late side effects (20).

A more rational approach to improving the selectivity of drugs for cancer therapy has been discussed by Bertino (2). Using folate antagonists as "prototype compounds," Bertino has reviewed the development of "rescue" agents, the potential sequence dependency of such combinations as methotrexate (MTX) and 5-fluorouracil (5-FU), new folate antagonists, and strategy for prevention of drug resistance.

The many factors that influence the results of chemotherapy are usually divided into three categories, relating to: the drug, the host, and the tumor (91,92). These factors interact significantly, and the planning of chemotherapy programs must keep them in mind.

Host factors include the physiologic and psychologic status of the patients. Drugs may suppress the immunologic interaction between host and tumor. The type, intensity, recency, tolerance, and result of prior treatment will influence significantly the nature and timing of subsequent chemotherapy. Among the tumor factors are the histopathology, biology, cellular kinetics, vascularization, extent of spread in the body, degree of sensitivities, and presence of anatomic sanctuaries. Drug factors include the metabolism and pharmacology of the drug, dose, and schedule of administration and manifestations of toxicity. Combinations and sequence of drugs are major considerations.

ABBREVIATIONS

Shorthand designation of a complex chemical name of a drug is common practice; unfortunately, however, no standard glossary exists. Abbreviations used in this chapter to indicate frequently administered agents are listed in Table 1.

CHEMOTHERAPEUTIC AGENTS

Table 2 lists the drugs that are being used relatively frequently in clinical pediatric oncology, with particular reference to malig-

TABLE 1. *Abbreviations for drugs*

Drug	Abbreviations used herein	Other abbreviations
Adriamycin	ADR	
Actinomycin D	AMD	Dact
1,3-bis(B-chloroethyl)-1-nitrosourea	BCNU	
Bleomycin	Bleo	
Citrovorum factor	CF	
Cyclophosphamide	CYT	CTX
cis-Platinum (II) diammine dichloride	DDP	Cisplatin CPDD
5-(3,3-dimethyl-triazene)-imidazole-4-carboxamide	DTIC	DIC
5-Fluorouracil	5-FU	FU
High-dose methotrexate	HD-MTX	
Methotrexate	MTX	
Nitrogen mustard	HN_2	
Phenylalanine mustard	PAM	
Vincristine	VCR	
Velban	VLB	

TABLE 2. Cancer chemotherapeutic agents used in childhood solid tumors

Drug	Route of adminis- tration	Usual dose	Major toxicity	Special conditions increasing risk of toxicity
Nitrogen mustard HN₂, Mustargen	i.v.	0.4 mg/kg	Severe nausea and vomiting Myelosuppression Acute contact vesicant Thrombophlebitis Marked tissue reaction on extravasation	
Chlorambucil Leukeran	p.o.	0.1 to 0.2 mg/kg/day	Cumulative myelosuppres- sion	
Cyclophosphamide Endoxan Cytoxan	i.v. p.o.	3.5 to 5.0 mg/kg/day × 10 5 to 10 mg/kg/day × 5 40 to 60 mg/kg/single dose 2.5 mg/kg daily	Myelosuppression Hemorrhagic cystitis Cardiomyopathy (after high doses) Gonadal dysfunction Antidiuretic effect	Infants Bladder irradiation Dehydration
High-dose methotrexate	i.v.	100 to 300 mg/kg as 4 to 6 hr drip, weekly or tri- weekly	Death Oral and GI ulceration Myelosuppression Renal damage Hepatic damage CNS toxicity	Renal dysfunction Hepatic dysfunction Inadequate hydration Acid urine Older children; 10 or more prior courses
5-Fluorouracil 5-FU fluorouracil	i.v. p.o.	300 to 400 mg/M²/day × 3 500 to 600 mg/M²/week	Stomatitis G-I ulceration Diarrhea Myelosuppression Reaction on extravasation	Hepatic dysfunction Hepatic irradiation

Drug	Route	Dose	Toxicity	Special precautions
Actinomycin D Cosmegen dactinomycin	i.v.	15 mcg/kg/day × 5 per course	Myelosuppression (especially thrombocytopenia) Nausea and vomiting Stomatitis Severe local tissue reaction on extravasation Irradiation sensitization	Infants Liver dysfunction Liver irradiation
Adriamycin doxorubicin	i.v.	45 to 75 mg/M^2 in single or divided doses over 2 to 3 days; repeat triweekly	Stomatitis Nausea and vomiting Myelosuppression Cardiomyopathy Severe local tissue reaction on extravasation Impaired wound healing (?)	Infants Cardiac irradiation Cumulative dose over 500 mg/M^2 Hepatic damage Heart disease
Bleomycin Blenoxane	i.v. i.m. s.q.	10 to 20 mg/M^2 1 to 2 ×/week	Hypotension Pyrexia Skin changes (micro-cutaneous ulceration) Pulmonary fibrosis	Cumulative dose over 200 mg/M^2 Prior or concurrent pulmonary irradiation
DTIC dacarbazine	i.v.	150 to 250 mg/M^2 day × 5	Marked nausea and vomiting Myelosuppression Local reaction on extravasation	Renal damage
BCNU carmustine	i.v.	100 to 200 mg/M^2 every 6 weeks	Nausea and vomiting Diarrhea Delayed and prolonged myelosuppression Nephrotoxicity Phlebitis	Rapid infusion

TABLE 2. *(Cont.)*

Drug	Route of administration	Usual dose	Major toxicity	Special conditions increasing risk of toxicity
cis-Platinum (II) diammine dichloride cisplatin	i.v. i.a.	(Dose still under study) 60 mg/M^2/day $\times$ 2 every 3 weeks	Severe nausea and vomiting Myelosuppression Renal damage Deafness Local reaction on extravasation	Dehydration Renal damage
Vincristine Oncovin	i.v.	1.5 to 2.0 mg/M^2 (maximum often 2 mg/dose)	Obstipation Severe abdominal pain Peripheral neuropathy Local tissue reaction on extravasation	Hepatic dysfunction Hepatic irradiation Infants
Vinblastine Velban	i.v.	4 to 6 mg/M^2/week	Myelosuppression Lethargy Peripheral neuropathy Local reaction on extravasation	Liver dysfunction

nant solid tumors. The routes of administration and the usual dosages are indicated. Dose-limiting major toxicities are given. In the final column are described situations requiring special caution. Preexisting organ dysfunctions, particularly if they affect the kidneys or the liver, will necessitate care in the administration of drugs that are damaging to either the kidneys or the liver. Drugs that are detoxified in the liver must be given with caution when irradiation includes the liver. Extravasation of such drugs as HN_2, ADR, daunomycin, AMD, and VCR can cause extremely painful tissue reaction, extensive ulceration, and sloughing. Intensive prior chemotherapy or irradiation of large bone marrow bearing areas may lead to severe and prolonged myelosuppression. Finally, the infant under 1 year of age may be susceptible to toxic effects of AMD, VCR, CYT, and ADR.

Other circumstances that may apply generally to all patients include extensive and intensive prior treatment (with reduction in bone marrow volume and regenerative capacity), widespread disease with bone marrow involvement, metastatic disease causing marked physiologic dysfunction, undernutrition, and presence of infection. Also, to be kept in mind constantly are the nature, extent, and intensity of other treatment modalities used concurrently.

Additional important information on cancer chemotherapeutic agents, including chemical name and structure, class of agent, mechanism of action, and cell cycle specificity, can be obtained from readily available sources (38,44,51,90,91).

STRATEGY OF CHEMOTHERAPY

Animal and laboratory data provide the bases for discussions of the conceptual aspects of the strategy for clinical cancer chemotherapy (2–4,14,15,54,63,76,89,90). The effectiveness of the strategies must be measured, ultimately, in terms of disease control and survival rates in patients with cancer. The magnitudes of disease control and survival rates in turn depend on the biologic sensitivity of the tumor to drug action and the selective effectiveness of the drug.

The objectives of chemotherapy parallel the overall objectives listed in the chapter on multimodal therapy. When considerations are limited specifically to chemotherapy, the objectives can be listed as follows:

1. Primary treatment with intent to cure. Chemotherapy is one component which with radiotherapy and/or surgery is expected to improve the probability of cure.
2. Secondary treatment of metastatic or recurrent tumor. Here, the purpose still can be curative ("retrieval") or, as is more generally the situation, to achieve meaningfully prolonged control of disease activity even though the disease returns.
3. Tertiary treatment of advanced disease to provide as much palliation as possible.

Tactically, chemotherapy can achieve these results in several ways, including:

1. Direct destruction of tumor cells and microscopic metastatic foci.
2. Reduction of tumor mass to facilitate surgical and/or radiotherapeutic attack.
3. Sensitization of tumor cells to antineoplastic action of other drugs (theoretical) or to irradiation (35); the synergism of AMD and irradiation is one example (23).
4. Participation in the "mopping up" process directed to residual tumor cells after major reduction in mass by another drug or modality.
5. Improving the effectiveness of the treatment program to permit refinement of therapy (omission of drug or modality, reduction in intensity).

COMBINATION CHEMOTHERAPY

The current trend in the management of most childhood solid tumors is the administration of combinations of chemotherapeutic agents (concurrently, sequentially, or alternately) instead of single agent therapy. The combinations are based on general principles, which have been summarized in several recent publications (2, 4,13,32,51,74,77). Krakoff (51) has outlined the various concepts: Use of drugs (a) that have antitumor activity when administered singly, (b) that have biochemical bases for possible synergism, (c) that have different mechanisms of action, (d) that have different patterns of major toxicity, i.e., affect different organ systems, (e) in which maximum toxicity occurs at different times after administration, to avoid cumulative toxicity, (f) in intermittent courses to minimze immunosuppression, and (g) each in full therapeutic dosage.

Through clinical usage, many combinations of drugs have acquired popular acronymic designations that identify them. Some of the more commonly administered combinations are shown on Table 3 along with indications and representative references. The same drug combination may be used in different studies, but the dosage and/or schedule may vary from one investigator to another. The reader should check the references for these details. It has been possible to include only a few of the many publications that pertain to combination chemotherapy in childhood solid tumors.

While the enhancement of therapeutic effect is the major objective of drug combination regimens, there exists the ominous possibility that the combinations may increase the risk of untoward side effects. For example, a high frequency of cardiomyopathy was reported after ADR had been combined with DTIC (9,80). In one trial, the occurrence of Pneumocystis carinii pneumonia was unusually frequent (9). The gonadal dysfunctions reported after treatment for Hodgkin's disease are particularly demonstrable among patients who received intensive chemotherapy (24,75).

ASSESSMENT OF THERAPEUTIC EFFECTIVENESS

The major chemotherapy regimens for the management of childhood solid tumors include the simultaneous or sequential

TABLE 3. *Drug combinations in clinical use*

Drugs in combination	Acronym	Clinical use	Refs.
VCR AMD CYT	VAC	Rhabdomyosarcoma Embryonal carcinoma Ovarian cancer Ewing's sarcoma Osteosarcoma	25,55,56,64,82 10,78,79 10,78,79 45,48,50,59,62 87
VCR AMD		Wilms' tumor Rhabdomyosarcoma	21,22 55,56
VCR CYT		Neuroblastoma Ewing's sarcoma	49 18,30
VCR AMD ADR		Wilms' tumor	21
VCR CYT ADR		Ewing's sarcoma Neuroblastoma	50,62 33
VCR AMD CYT ADR	T-2	Rhabdomyosarcoma Ewing's sarcoma	29,34 65,66,71
VCR CYT ADR 5-FU	AD-CON-FU	Rhabdomyosarcoma Neuroblastoma Embryonal carcinoma Lymphoepithelioma	8 8 8 8
VCR CYT Procarbazine Papaverine		Neuroblastoma	42,43,61
AMD 5-FU CYT	ACT-FU-CY	Embryonal carcinoma Ovarian cancer	78,79 78,79
ADR DTIC	Adria-DIC	Various solid tumors Ewing's tumor Neuroblastoma	9,37 9 9,52
CYT VCR AMD DTIC	CY-VA-DIC	Sarcomas (especially in adults)	36

TABLE 3. *(Cont.)*

Drugs in combination	Acronym	Clinical use	Refs.
VCR HD-MTX ADR		Osteosarcoma	47,68
BLEO CYT AMD	BCD	Osteosarcoma (metastatic)	58
CYT VCR PAM ADR	CONPADRI	Osteosarcoma	84,85
ADR DDP		Osteosarcoma	28
CYT VCR HD-MTX PAM ADR	COMPADRI	Osteosarcoma	85,86
HD-MTX CYT ADR VCR	T-4, T-5	Osteosarcoma	67,70
VCR AMD CYT MTX BLEO ADR BCNU	T-6	Rhabdomyosarcoma Ewing's sarcoma	29 66
VCR AMD CYT BLEO HD-MTX ADR	T-7	Osteosarcoma	68,69
VLB BLEO		Testicular cancer Germ cell cancer	72,73 72,73
VLB BLEO DDP	PVB	Testicular cancer	27

TABLE 3. *(Cont.)*

Drugs in combination	Acronym	Clinical use	Refs.
VCR BLEO ADR		Testicular cancer	6
VCR BLEO CYT MTX 5-FU		Testicular cancer	72
HN$_2$ VCR Procarbazine Prednisone	MOPP	Brain tumor	11
VCR BCNU Dexamethasone MTX		Brain tumor	26,88
VCR CYT DTIC		Neuroblastoma	31,39
VCR ADR HN$_2$ DTIC		Neuroblastoma	46
VCR CYT HN$_2$		Neuroblastoma	46

use of drugs in combinations. When two or more drugs are administered together, the combined antitumor activity may indeed be additive or possibly synergistic. For example, when VCR and AMD are given as adjuvant chemotherapy, the survival rates are significantly better than those attained by either drug alone (22). The clinical effectiveness of the three-drug combination of VAC (Table 3) is significantly better than the results obtained by any one of the drugs used singly in rhabdomyosarcoma (25,82). Therefore, less than maximum performance during single-agent therapeutic trials does not exclude the potential usefulness of the agent when administered in combination. Conversely, the component drugs of an effective combination should not be expected to yield equal activity when used singly. For background

TABLE 4. *Effectiveness of single-agent chemotherapy in specific tumors*

Tumor	Drugs with major activity	Drugs with minor but definite activity
Wilms' tumor	AMD VCR ADR	CYT
Osteosarcoma	HD-MTX ADR DDP	PAM
Rhabdomyosarcoma	VCR CYT ADR	AMD
Neuroblastoma	CYT VCR AMD Peptichemio	DDP DTIC
Ewing's sarcoma	CYT ADR	VCR AMD
Brain tumors		VCR Procarbazine HD-MTX Nitrosourea
Germ cell tumors	VLB BLEO DDP	AMD VCR CYT 5-FU
Carcinomas		5-FU ADR
Hepatoma		AMD ADR

information, the basic assessment of the effectiveness of single-agent chemotherapy in specific tumors has been tabulated (Table 4). Drug combinations are discussed in another section of this chapter.

The major solid tumor categories in children are listed in Table 4. The drugs used for each tumor are divided into two columns, depending on expected effectiveness. Drugs listed as possessing major activity will have produced objective responses fairly regularly in metastatic situations and will have been used effectively in the primary treatment of the tumor. Drugs listed as possessing minor activity are those that produce responses less consistently and often of lesser degree (partial regressions rather than complete responses).

Although improvement in survival rates and disease control has been demonstrated in such cancers as Wilms' tumor, osteosarcoma, and rhabdomyosarcoma, the assessment of the contribution of chemotherapy alone to the results of multimodal programs is difficult. However, Table 5 considers aspects of cancer therapy where some evaluation might be possible.

First is the documentation of improved cure rates. Second, the prolongation of disease control can be measured as duration of disease-free survival and overall survival. Third, the usefulness of drugs in postmetastatic treatment can be measured by the response of the metastatic disease, by the rate of postmetastatic retrievals (cures), and by the duration of postmetastatic survival. The fourth aspect takes into account not only the availability of adjuvant regimens in nonmetastatic cases but also evidence that such adjuvant programs have yielded positive data (improved survival).

TABLE 5. Assessment of chemotherapy contribution to results of treatment

Tumor	Improved cure rate	Prolongation of disease control	Useful post-metastatic treatment	Effective adjuvant program for nonmetastatic cases
Wilms' tumor	Yes	Yes	Yes	Yes
Osteosarcoma	Probably	Yes	Yes	Yes
Rhabdomyosarcoma	Yes	Yes	Yes	Yes
Ewing's sarcoma	Probably	Probably	Yes	Yes
Neuroblastoma	Not established	Possibly	Yes	To be demonstrated
Brain tumors	Not established	Possibly	Yes	Same
Ovarian cancer	Possibly	Yes	Yes	Same
Testicular cancer	Possibly	Yes	Yes	Same
Carcinomas	No	Possibly	Probably	Not demonstrated

REFERENCES

1. Becker, F. F. (editor) (1977): *Cancer—A Comprehensive Treatise, Vol. 5.* Plenum, New York.
2. Bertino, J. R. (1979): Toward improved selectivity in cancer chemotherapy: The Richard and Hinda Rosenthal Foundation Award Lecture. *Cancer Res.,* 39:293–304.
3. Block, J. B., and Isacoff, W. H. (1977): Adjuvant chemotherapy in cancer. *Semin. Oncol.,* 4:109–115.
4. Brady, L. W., and Markoe, A. M. (1979): The biologic basis for combined modality treatment of cancer. *Cancer Clin. Trials,* 2:5–18.
5. Burchenal, J. H. (1977): The historical development of cancer chemotherapy. *Semin. Oncol.,* 4:135–146.
6. Burgess, M. A., Einhorn, L. H., and Gottlieb, J. A. (1977): Treatment of metastatic germ-cell tumors in men with adriamycin, vincristine, and bleomycin. *Cancer Treat. Rep.,* 61:1447–1451.
7. *Cancer Chemotherapy. Fundamental Concepts and Recent Advances* (1975): Year Book Medical Publishers, Chicago.
8. Cangir, A., Falletta, J. M., Ragab, A. H., and McMillan, C. (1978): Combination chemotherapy with adriamycin, cyclophosphamide, vincristine, and 5-fluorouracil (AD-CON-FU) in children with metastatic solid tumors and untreated rare tumors. *Proc. AACR ASCO,* 19:391 (Abstr.).
9. Cangir, A., Morgan, S. K., Land, V. J., Pullen, J., Starling, K. A., and Nitschke, R. (1976): Combination chemotherapy with adriamycin and dimethyl triazeno imidazole carboxamide (DTIC) in children with metastatic solid tumors. *Med. Pediatr. Oncol.,* 2:183–190.
10. Cangir, A., Smith, J., and van Eys, J. (1978): Improved prognosis in children with ovarian cancers following modified VAC (vincristine sulfate, dactinomycin, and cyclophosphamide) chemotherapy. *Cancer,* 42:1234–1238.
11. Cangir, A., van Eys, J., Berry, D. H., Hvizdula, E., and Morgan, S. K. (1978): Combination chemotherapy with MOPP in children with recurrent brain tumors. *Med. Pediatr. Oncol.,* 4:253–261.
12. Capizzi, R. L. (editor) (1977): The pharmacologic basis of cancer chemotherapy. *Semin. Oncol.,* 4:131–262.
13. Capizzi, R. L., Keiser, L. W., and Sartorelli, A. C. (1977): Combination chemotherapy—theory and practice. *Semin. Oncol.,* 4:227–253.
14. Carter, S. K. (1974): Integration of chemotherapy into combined modality treatment of solid tumors. 1. The overall strategy. *Cancer Treat. Rev.,* 1:1–18.
15. Carter, S. K. (1977): The strategy of cancer treatment: Introduction. *Recent Results Cancer Res.,* 62:51–55.
16. Chabner, B. A., Myers, C. E., Coleman, C. N., and Johns, D. V. (1975): The clinical pharmacology of antineoplastic agents. *N. Engl. J. Med.,* 292:1107–1113, 1159–1168.
17. Chabner, B. A., Myers, C. E., and Oliverio, V. T. (1977): Clinical pharmacology of anticancer drugs. *Semin. Oncol.,* 4:165–191.
18. Chan, R. C., Sutow, W. W., Lindberg, R. D., Samuels, M. L., Murray,

J. A., and Johnston, D. A. (1979): Management and results of localized Ewing's sarcoma. *Cancer,* 43:1001–1006.

19. Clarysse, A., Kenis, Y., and Mathe, G. (editors) (1976): Cancer chemotherapy. *Recent Results Cancer Res.,* 53:1–566.

20. Creaven, P. J., and Mihich, E. (1977): The clinical toxicity of anticancer drugs and its prediction. *Semin. Oncol.,* 4:147–163.

21. D'Angio, G. J., Beckwith, J. B., Breslow, N., Sinks, L., Sutow, W. W., and Wolff, J. (1979): Results of the second National Wilms' Tumor Study (NWTS-2). *Proc. AACR ASCO,* 20:309 (Abstr.).

22. D'Angio, G. J., Evans, A. E., Breslow, N., Beckwith, B., Bishop, H., Feigl, P., Goodwin, W., Leape, L. L., Sinks, L. F., Sutow, W., Tefft, M., and Wolff, J. (1976): The treatment of Wilms' tumor. Results of the National Wilms' Tumor Study. *Cancer,* 38:633–646.

23. D'Angio, G. J., Maddock, C. L., Farber, S., and Brown, B. L. (1965): The enhanced response of the Ridgway osteogenic sarcoma to roentgen radiation combined with actinomycin D. *Cancer Res.,* 25:1002–1007.

24. De Vita, V. T., Arsenau, J. C., Sherins, R. J., Canellos, G. P., and Young R. C. (1973): Intensive chemotherapy for Hodgkin's disease: Long-term complications. *Natl. Cancer Inst. Monogr.,* 36:447–454.

25. Donaldson, S. S., Castro, J. R., Wilbur, J. R., and Jesse, R. H. (1973): Rhabdomyosarcoma of head and neck in children—combination treatment by surgery, irradiation, and chemotherapy. *Cancer,* 31:26–35.

26. Duffner, P. K., Cohen, M. E., Thomas, P. R. M., Sinks, L. F., and Freeman, A. I. (1979): Combination chemotherapy in recurrent medulloblastoma. *Cancer,* 43:41–45.

27. Einhorn, L. H., and Donahue, J. (1977): cis-Diamminedichloroplatinum, vinblastine, and bleomycin combination chemotherapy in disseminated testicular cancer. *Ann. Intern. Med.,* 87:293–298.

28. Ettinger, L. J., Douglass, H. O., Jr., Higby, D. J., Nime, F., Bjornsson, S., Mindell, E. R., Ghoorah, J., Freeman, A. I., and Moskowitz, R. M. (1979): Adriamycin and cis-diamminedichloroplatinum as adjuvant therapy in primary osteosarcoma. *Proc. AACR ASCO,* 20:438 (Abstr.).

29. Exelby, P. R., Ghavimi, F., and Jereb, B. (1978): Genitourinary rhabdomyosarcoma in children. *J. Pediatr. Surg.,* 13:746–752.

30. Fernandez, C. H., Lindberg, R. D., Sutow, W. W., and Samuels, M. L. (1974): Localized Ewing's sarcoma: Treatment and results. *Cancer,* 34:143–148.

31. Finklestein, J. Z., Leikin, S., Evans, A., Klemperer, M., Bernstein, I., Hittle, R., and Hammond, G. D. (1974): Combination chemotherapy for metastatic neuroblastoma. *Proc. AACR ASCO,* 15:44 (Abstr.).

32. Frei, E., III (1972): Combination chemotherapy. *Cancer Res.,* 32:2593–2607.

33. Gasparini, M., Bellani, F. F., Musumeci, R., and Bonadonna, G. (1974): Response and survival of patients with metastatic neuroblastoma after combination chemotherapy with adriamycin, cyclophosphamide, and vincristine. *Cancer Chemother. Rep.,* 58:365–370.

34. Ghavimi, F., Exelby, P. R., D'Angio, G. J., Cham, W., Lieberman, P. H.,

Tan, C., Miké, V., and Murphy, M. L. (1975): Multidisciplinary treatment of embryonal rhabdomyosarcoma in children. *Cancer,* 36:677–686.

35. Goffinet, D. R., and Bagshaw, M. A. (1974): Clinical use of radiation sensitizing agents. *Cancer Treat. Rev.,* 1:15–26.

36. Gottlieb, J. A., Baker, L. H., Burgess, M. A., Sinkovics, J. G., Moon T., Bodey, G. P., Rodriguez, V., Rivkin, S. E., Saiki, J., and O'Bryan, R. M. (1975): Sarcoma chemotherapy. In: *Cancer Chemotherapy. Fundamental Concepts and Recent Advances,* pp. 445–454. Year Book Medical Publishers, Chicago.

37. Gottlieb, J. A., Baker, L. H., Quagliana, J. M., Luce, J. K., Whitecar, J. P., Jr., Sinkovics, J. G., Rivkin, S. E., Brownlee, R., and Frei, E., III (1972): Chemotherapy of sarcomas with a combination of adriamycin and dimethyl triazeno imidazole carboxamide. *Cancer,* 30:1632–1638.

38. Greenspan, E. M. (editor) (1975): *Clinical Cancer Chemotherapy.* Raven Press, New York.

39. Grosfeld, J. L., Schatzlein, M., Ballantine, T. V., Weetman, R. M., and Baehner, R. L. (1978): Metastatic neuroblastoma: Factors influencing survival. *J. Pediatr. Surg.,* 13:59–65.

40. Hall, T. C. (1971): Prediction of response in cancer therapy. *Natl. Cancer Inst. Monogr.,* 34:1–298.

41. Hall, T. C. (1977): Prediction of responses to therapy and mechanisms of resistance. *Semin. Oncol.,* 4:193–202.

42. Helson, L. (1975): Management of disseminated neuroblastoma. *CA,* 25:264–277.

43. Helson, L., Helson, C., Peterson, R. F., and Das, S. K. (1976): A rationale for the treatment of metastatic neuroblastoma. *J. Natl. Cancer Inst.,* 57:727–729.

44. Holland, J. F., and Frei, E., III (editors) (1973): The chemotherapeutic agents. In: *Cancer Medicine,* section XIII, pp. 739–888. Lea & Febiger, Philadelphia.

45. Hustu, H. O., Pinkel, D., and Pratt, C. B. (1972): Treatment of clinically localized Ewing's sarcoma with radiotherapy and combination chemotherapy. *Cancer,* 30:1522–1527.

46. Jaffe, N. (1976): Neuroblastoma: Review of the literature and an examination of factors contributing to its enigmatic character. *Cancer Treat. Rev.,* 3:61–82.

47. Jaffe, N., and Traggis, D. (1975): Toxicity of high-dose methotrexate and citrovorum factor in osteogenic sarcoma. *Cancer Chemother. Rep.,* Part 3. 6:31–36.

48. Jaffe, N., Traggis, D., Salian, S., and Cassady, J. R. (1976): Improved outlook for Ewing's sarcoma with combination chemotherapy (vincristine, actinomycin D, and cyclophosphamide) and radiation therapy. *Cancer,* 38:1925–1930.

49. James, D. H., Jr., Hustu, O., Wrenn, E. L., Jr., and Pinkel, D. (1965): Combination chemotherapy of childhood neuroblastoma. *JAMA,* 194:123–126.

50. Johnson, R. E., and Pomeroy, T. C. (1975): Evaluation of therapeutic results in Ewing's sarcoma. *Am. J. Roentgenol. Rad. Ther. Nucl. Med.*, 123:583–587.
51. Krakoff, I. H. (1977): Cancer chemotherapeutic agents. *CA*, 27:130–143.
52. Leikin, S., Bernstein, I., Evans, A., Finklestein, J., Hittle, R., and Klemperer, M. (1978): Use of combination adriamycin and DTIC in children with advanced stage IV neuroblastoma. *Cancer Chemother. Rep.*, 59:1015–1018.
53. Livingston, R. B., and Carter, S. K. (1970): *Single Agents in Cancer Chemotherapy.* Plenum, New York.
54. Mathe, G. (editor) (1977): Tactics and strategy in cancer treatment. *Recent Results Cancer Treat.*, 62:1–219.
55. Maurer, H. M., Donaldson, M., Gehan, E. A., Hammond, D., Hays, D. M., Lawrence, W., Jr., Lindberg, R., Newton, W., Ragab, A., Raney, R. B., Ruymann, F., Soule, E. II., Sutow, W. W., and Tefft, M. (1980): The Intergroup Rhabdomyosarcoma Study—update November 1978. *Natl. Cancer Inst. Monogr. (in press).*
56. Maurer, H. M., Moon, T., Donaldson, M., Fernandez, C., Gehan, E. A., Hammond, D., Hays, D. M., Lawrence, W., Jr., Newton, W., Ragab, A., Raney, B., Soule, E. H., Sutow, W. W., and Tefft, M. (1977): The Intergroup Rhabdomyosarcoma Study. A preliminary report. *Cancer*, 40:2015–2026.
57. Mihich, E. (1973): Pharmacologic principles and the basis for selectivity of drug action. In: *Cancer Medicine,* edited by J. F. Holland and E. Frei, III, pp. 650–674. Lea & Febiger, Philadelphia.
58. Mosende, C., Gutierrez, M., Caparros, B., and Rosen, G. (1977): Combination chemotherapy with bleomycin, cyclophosphamide, and dactinomycin for the treatment of osteogenic sarcoma. *Cancer*, 40:2779–2786.
59. Nesbit, M. E., Perez, C. A., Tefft, M., Burgert, E. O., Vietti, T. J., Kissane, J., Pritchard, D., and Gehan, E. A. (1980): Multimodal therapy for the management of primary, nonmetastatic Ewing's sarcoma of bone: An intergroup study. *Natl. Cancer Inst. Monogr. (in press).*
60. Nichol, C. A. (1977): Pharmacokinetics. Selectivity of action related to physiochemical properties and kinetic patterns of anticancer drugs. *Cancer,* 40:519–528.
61. Nitschke, R., Cangir, A., Crist, W., and Berry, D. H. (1979): Intensive chemotherapy for metastatic neuroblastoma, Southwest Oncology Group Study. *Proc. AACR ASCO,* 20:392 (Abstr.).
62. Pomeroy, T. C., and Johnson, R. E. (1975): Combined modality therapy of Ewing's sarcoma. *Cancer,* 35:36–47.
63. Proceedings of the Symposium on Cell Kinetics and Cancer Chemotherapy (Annapolis, Maryland, November 4–6, 1975) (1976): *Cancer Treat. Rep.,* 60:1697–1979.
64. Raney, R. B., Jr., Gehan, E. A., Maurer, H. M., Newton, W. A. Jr., Ragab, A. H., Ruymann, F. B., Sutow, W. W., and Tefft, M. (1979): Evaluation of intensified chemotherapy in children with advanced rhabdomyosarcoma (clinical Groups III and IV). *Cancer Clin. Trials,* 2:19–28.

65. Rosen, G. (1977): Past experiences and future considerations with T-2 chemotherapy in the treatment of Ewing's sarcoma. In: *Management of Primary Bone and Soft Tissue Tumors,* pp. 187–203. Year Book Medical Publishers, Chicago.

66. Rosen, G., Caparros, B., Mosende, C., McCormick, B., Huvos, A. G., and Marcove, R. C. (1978): Curability of Ewing's sarcoma and considerations for future therapeutic trials. *Cancer,* 41:888–899.

67. Rosen, G., Huvos, A. G., Mosende, C., Beattie, E. J., Jr., Exelby, P. R., Capparos, B., and Marcove, R. C. (1978): Chemotherapy and thoracotomy for metastatic osteogenic sarcoma. A model for adjuvant chemotherapy and the rationale for timing of thoracic surgery. *Cancer,* 41:841–849.

68. Rosen, G., and Jaffe, N. (1979): Chemotherapy of malignant spindle cell sarcomas of bone. In: *Bone Tumors in Children,* edited by N. Jaffe, pp. 107–130. PSG Publishing, Littleton, Massachusetts.

69. Rosen, G., Marcove, R. C., Caparros, B., Nirenberg, A., Kosloff, C., and Huvos, A. G. (1980): Primary osteogenic sarcoma: The rationale for preoperative chemotherapy and delayed surgery. *Natl. Cancer Inst. Monogr. (in press).*

70. Rosen, G., Murphy, M. L., Huvos, A. G., Gutierrez, M., and Marcove, R. C. (1976): Chemotherapy, en bloc resection, and prosthetic replacement in the treatment of osteogenic sarcoma. *Cancer,* 37:1–11.

71. Rosen, G., Wollner, N., Tan, C., Wu, S. T., Hadju, S. I., Cham, W., D'Angio, G. J., and Murphy, M. L. (1974): Disease-free survival in children with Ewing's sarcoma treated with radiation therapy and adjuvant four-drug sequential chemotherapy. *Cancer,* 33:384–393.

72. Samuels, M. L., Holoye, P. Y., and Johnson, D. E. (1975): Bleomycin combination chemotherapy in the management of testicular neoplasia. *Cancer,* 36:318–326.

73. Samuels, M. L., Lanzotti, V. J., Holoye, P. Y., Boyle, L. E., Smith, T. L., and Johnson, D. E. (1976): Combination chemotherapy of germinal cell tumors. *Cancer Treat. Rev.,* 3:185–204.

74. Sartorelli, A. C., and Creasy, W. A. (1973): Combination chemotherapy. In: *Cancer Medicine,* edited by J. F. Holland and E. Frei, III, pp. 707–716. Lea & Febiger, Philadelphia.

75. Sherins, R. J., Olweny, C. L. M., and Ziegler, J. L. (1978): Gynecomastia and gonadal dysfunction in adolescent boys treated with combination chemotherapy for Hodgkin's disease. *N. Engl. J. Med.,* 299:12–16.

76. Skipper, H. (1968): Biochemical, biological, pharmacologic, toxicologic, kinetic, and clinical (subhuman and human) relationships. *Cancer,* 22:600.

77. Skipper, H. E. (1978): Adjuvant chemotherapy. *Cancer,* 41:936–940.

78. Smith, J. P. (1977): Malignant gynecologic tumors. In: *Clinical Pediatric Oncology,* second edition, edited by W. W. Sutow, T. J. Vietti, and D. J. Fernbach, pp. 654–663. C. V. Mosby, St. Louis.

79. Smith, J. P., Rutledge, F., and Sutow, W. W. (1973): Maliganant gynecologic tumors in children: Current approaches to treatment. *Am. J. Obstet. Gynecol.,* 116:261–270.

80. Smith, P. J., Ekert, H., Waters, K. D., and Matthews, R. N. (1977): High incidence of cardiomyopathy in children treated with adriamycin and DTIC in combination chemotherapy. *Cancer Treat. Rep.,* 61:1736–1738.
81. Sutow, W. W. (1965): Chemotherapy in childhood cancer (except leukemia). An appraisal. *Cancer,* 18:1585–1589.
82. Sutow, W. W. (1969): Chemotherapeutic management of childhood rhabdomyosarcoma. In: *Neoplasia in Childhood,* pp. 201–208. Year Book Medical Publishers, Chicago.
83. Sutow, W. W. (1975): Chemotherapy in the management of childhood solid tumors. In: *Cancer Chemotherapy. Fundamental Concepts and Recent Advances,* pp. 203–214. Year Book Medical Publishers, Chicago.
84. Sutow, W. W., Gehan, E. A., Dyment, P. G., Vietti, T., and Miale, T. (1978): Multidrug adjuvant chemotherapy for osteosarcoma: Interim report of the Southwest Oncology Group Studies. *Cancer Treat. Rep.,* 62:265–269.
85. Sutow, W. W., Gehan, E. A., Vietti, T. J., Frias, A. E., and Dyment, P. G. (1976): Multidrug chemotherapy in primary treatment of osteosarcoma. *J. Bone Joint Surg.,* 58-A:629–633.
86. Sutow, W. W., Sullivan, M. P., Fernbach, D. J., Cangir, A., and George, S. L. (1975): Adjuvant chemotherapy in primary treatment of osteogenic sarcoma. *Cancer,* 36:1598–1602.
87. Sutow, W. W., Sullivan, M. P., Wilbur, J. R., and Cangir, A. (1975): Study of adjuvant chemotherapy in osteogenic sarcoma. *J. Clin. Pharmacol.,* 15:530–533.
88. Thomas, P. R. M., Duffner, P. K., Cohen, M. E., Sinks, L. F., and Freeman, A. I. (1979): Multimodality therapy for medulloblastoma. *Proc. AACR ASCO,* 20:325 (Abstr.).
89. Valeriote, F. A., and Edelstein, M. B. (1977): The role of cell kinetics in cancer chemotherapy. *Semin. Oncol.,* 4:217–226.
90. Valeriote, F., and Vietti, T. J. (1977): Cellular kinetics and conceptual basis of chemotherapy. In: *Clinical Pediatric Oncology,* second edition, edited by W. W. Sutow, T. J. Vietti, and D. J. Fernbach, pp. 182–196. C. V. Mosby, St. Louis.
91. Vietti, T. J., Valeriote, F., and Mutz, I. D. (1977): General aspects of chemotherapy. In: *Clinical Pediatric Oncology,* second edition, edited by W. W. Sutow, T. J. Vietti, and D. J. Fernbach, pp. 197–237. C. V. Mosby, St. Louis.
92. Zubrod, C. G. (1978): Selective toxicity of anticancer drugs: Presidential address. *Cancer Res.,* 38:4377–4384.

5

Neuroblastoma

Neuroblastoma, the maverick tumor, manifests a puzzlingly upredictable biologic behavior and remains a major therapeutic frustration in pediatric oncology.

LITERATURE SCAN

In 1959, Gross et al. (41) published a comprehensive report on neuroblastoma and emphasized some important observations:

1. Neuroblastoma was a relatively frequent malignant solid tumor in children.
2. The younger children, particularly infants less than 1 year of age, had a markedly better outlook for survival than older children.
3. The presence of skeletal metastases had an extremely serious prognostic significance; practically all such patients died.
4. The survival pattern in neuroblastoma suggested that the site of the primary tumor may be correlated with survival. Tumors of adrenal and abdominal sympathetic origin had the poorest survival.
5. The occurrence of spontaneous regression of the tumor was noted in some patients.
6. Patients with liver metastases were frequently "cured."

These authors thought that multimodal therapy (surgery plus radiotherapy) had improved the survival rate. They concluded with an optimistic prediction: "Impressive changes clearly give a bright hope that in the future significant improvements in therapy for neuroblastoma will come from the chemotherapeutic attacks" (41).

The status of the neuroblastoma question was reexamined at a conference on the biology of neuroblastoma held in 1967 (7). From the surgeon's viewpoint, Koop (55) noted "a lack of correlation between the survival of the patient and the mode of surgical therapy." A cautious question was also voiced regarding the actual usefulness of radiation therapy in these children other than for palliative purposes (54).

It was pointed out that most of the basic requirements for potentially curative chemotherapy can be met in neuroblastoma: (a) a chemosensitive tumor, (b) availability of relatively effective chemical agents, and (c) availability of other effective treatment modalities (89). However, no firm data indicated any improvement in survival as the result of added chemotherapy, and no effective adjuvant regimens were described. At the end of the conference, Schweisguth (83) observed succinctly that "prognosis in neuroblastoma seems related, more than to the type of treatment, to some unknown factors concerning the host and the tumor."

Another conference on neuroblastoma was held by the Société Internationale d'Oncologie Pédiatrique (SIOP) in October 1973 (85). Perusal of the papers suggests that no major advances were reported.

The Journal of the National Cancer Institute published the papers that had been presented 1 year previously (94). Helson et al. (45) outlined a four-drug treatment program which included, in addition to vincristine (VCR) and cyclophosphamide, papaverine and 5-trifluoromethyl-2'-deoxyuridine (F3TDR). The concept of "promoting maturation" by means of drugs was intriguing.

In 1976, a multiauthored monograph edited by Pochedly (74) discussed various aspects of neuroblastoma. The intent of the volume was "to organize the extensive literature on neuroblastoma into a workable and easily understood scheme." Recently, Jaffe (49) reviewed the literature covering numerous facets of neuroblastoma and characterized the tumor as having an "enigmatic character." In another review, Finkelstein (32) referred to neuroblastoma as a "unique solid tumor of childhood."

An examination of the many recent reports on neuroblastoma generates a grim awareness of a strong consensus that "the results of treatment have been disappointing" and that "the overall survival rate is the same today as it was prior to the use of chemotherapy" (25). In 1958, data from a literature survey (88) gave an overall survival rate (at 14 months) of 22% (103/450). In 1970, an analysis of questionnaire information from a nationwide survey (92) showed no significant improvement in overall survival between 84 children treated in 1956 and 142 children treated in 1962. In 1956, no effective drugs, other than the nitrogen mustards, were being used clinically. By 1962, actinomycin D and cyclophosphamide had become available. This type of analysis was extended in 1974 to include data on patients treated by the Children's Cancer Study Group A between 1966 and 1968 (64).

Although the patients in the study received intensive VCR and cyclophosphamide, comparisons with data from similar types of patients (with advanced disease) treated in previous years showed no change in survival.

Nonetheless, the published data can be tabulated in several ways to emphasize the recognition of certain patient and tumor characteristics as having prognostic significance. Such factors include (a) age of the patient at diagnosis, (b) anatomic site of the primary tumor, (c) extent of the disease in the patient (clinical stage), and (d) special stage IV-S category.

The major part of this chapter is concerned with the factors listed above. Numerous other aspects of the neuroblastoma problem are being investigated, but the impact of all the activities has not yet been reflected in improved overall survival statistics.

Several systems for histopathologic grading of neuroblastomas have been proposed (2,47,48). Beckwith and Martin (2) found a definite correlation between the degree of differentiation (maturation) and prognosis. Thus only 4% of 28 patients with grade IV undifferentiated tumors survived (2). In addition, the more differentiated types occurred more commonly in the younger children (2).

Hughes et al. (48) reported that a high level of histologic differentiation (grade) correlated with good survival and also with younger age and more favorable clinical stage.

The presence of lymphoid infiltrates has also been correlated with better prognosis (61,68). Statistical analyses have shown a significant quantitative relationship between degree of lymphoid infiltration and duration of survival (61,68). These correlations seemed to exist independent of the presence or absence of metastases. Hughes et al. (48), however, did not find a significant relationship between the degree of lymphocytic infiltration and prognosis.

Spontaneous regression of neuroblastoma has long been recognized clinically (15,27,30,82), and efforts have been made to study how this phenomenon may relate to the biology of the tumor (10,15,82). Beckwith and Perrin (3) reported neuroblastoma *in situ* in necropsy specimens of infants under 3 months of age dying of unrelated causes. The rate was estimated to be 40 times the expected incidence. The authors calculated that "of every 100 to 300 young infants coming to necropsy, 1 will be found to harbor a small, clinically unsuspected neuroblastoma" (3). Marsden and Steward (67) extended the calculations to postulate that "39 out of every 40 neuroblastomas present at birth regress spontaneously." The possible relationship of nerve growth factor (NGF) to maturation of neuroblastoma has also been studied (11,69); none has yet been demonstrated (8,59).

The immunology of neuroblastoma has also been subjected to extensive investigations (4–6,42), but the role of immunotherapy remains to be established (5,6). One preliminary study has suggested that the addition of nonspecific immunostimulatory agent (MER/BCG) to three-drug chemotherapy (VCR, adriamycin, and cyclophosphamide) prolonged the median duration of complete regression in 11 patients with stages III and IV neuroblastoma (70).

Biochemical studies in neuroblastoma represent another area of continued investigations, particularly as they relate to urinary catecholamine and amino acid patterns, both for diagnostic purposes and in their potential use as prognostic determinants (9,

40,60,74,98). Recently, Laug et al. (62) have reported that "the presence of the dopa metabolite, vanillactic acid, as well as increased amounts of cystathione and/or low levels of VMA indicated poor prognosis."

DATA SOURCE

Most of the data for the various tables in this chapter were compiled from the publications listed in Table 1. Care was exercised to minimize the use of overlapping data from institutions reporting independently as well as collaboratively. Separate reports from the same institution frequently contained additional information that was utilized in different tables for this chapter.

TABLE 1. *Data source for neuroblastoma*

Ref.	Institutions	Time	No. of patients	Nature of report
36	Memorial Hospital (NYC)	1951–1961	133	Patient characteristics
101	Villejuif (France)	1950–1970	390	Detailed study of survival and
	Amsterdam	1950–1970	72	patient characteristics
20	Children's Hospital of Philadelphia (CHOP)	1942–1974	181	Summary data on patient characteristics
12	CHOP	1947–1967	134	Statistical analysis of sur-
	Children's Cancer Study Group	1966–1968	112	vival and prognostic factors
52	Great Britain	1962–1967	487	Detailed study of survival and patient characteristics
49	Sidney Farber Cancer Center (SFCC)	Through 1975	267	Review of literature and inclusion of summary data from SFCC

Publications including data on more than 100 patients were selected whenever possible.

The substantial experience with neuroblastoma at the Children's Hospital has been reported at various times by different members of the clinical team. The surgical viewpoints have been expressed by Koop (54–56), Koop and Johnson (57), Gerson and Koop (38), Koop and Schnaufer (58), and Duckett and Koop (20). The same series provided the basic data for the development of the widely used staging schema (16,26) and for the statistical analyses of data utilizing this staging technique (12). The overall management and chemotherapy for these cases have been discussed periodically, including reports by Gerson and Koop (38) and by Evans et al. (25). The correlation of degree of maturation and differentiation with prognosis for survival was reported in 1956 by Horn et al. (47).

INCIDENCE

The estimate for incidence of neuroblastoma calculated from the data (Third National Cancer Survey) published by Young and Miller (100) is shown in Table 2. The incidence rates published from the SEER program (99) are about the same: 9.4 for whites and 6.7 for blacks per million population per year. Among the white children, neuroblastoma is the second most frequent malignant solid tumor, next to tumors of the central

TABLE 2. *Incidence of neuroblastoma and ganglioneuroblastoma in children in the United States[a]*

Race	Male	Female	Total	Percent of all solid tumors
White	5.4	4.1	9.5	13.7
Black	4.8	2.2	7.0	11.8

[a] Rate per million population per year calculated from data of Young and Miller (100).

nervous system (CNS) (99,100). Among the black children, neu-roblastoma ranks third in frequency, next to CNS tumors and Wilms tumor.

AGE

Age Distribution

Age of the patient at diagnosis has been one of the earliest host characteristics to be correlated with survival. The younger children had significantly better survival than the older children (12,19,41,88,92). For statistical considerations, the younger children were frequently defined as those younger than 14 or 24 months. Breslow and McCann (12) have shown that the age effect on survival was apparent in all clinical stages, and that the effect was most prominent during the first 2 years of life. After 2 years of age, the age effect tapered off. The analysis also showed that both age and stage remained important factors, even after adjusting for the effects of the other (12). Because of these considerations, tables have been prepared below to show the age distribution among published series and the relationship of age to clinical stage and site of primary tumor.

The age distribution has been derived from three different series in Table 3. Only slight variations occurred among the three series:

TABLE 3. *Age distribution in neuroblastoma*

| | Age (years) | | | | | | |
| | Under 1 | | 1 to 2 | | Over 2 | | Patient total |
Ref.	No.	%[a]	No.	%	No.	%	
101	143	31.0	85	18.4	234	50.6	462
52	121	24.8	79	16.2	287	58.9	487
12	69	28.0	47	19.1	130	52.8	246
	333	27.9	211	17.7	651	54.5	1,195

[a] Percent of patient total for the particular series.

27.9% of the combined total (1,195 patients) were under 1 year of age, 17.7% between 1 and 2 years, and 54.5% over 2 years. Thus less than one-half (45.6%) were in the prognostically favorable groups (under 2 years of age).

In a single institutional report, Jaffe (49) reported that among 321 patients seen at the Sidney Farber Cancer Center, the age distribution was 26.5% under 1 year, 17.4% from 1 to 2 years, and 56.1% over 2 years. A questionnaire survey conducted among the Surgical Fellows of the American Academy of Pediatrics (1) provided information on 573 cases of neuroblastoma seen between 1955 and 1965. According to the survey, 37.5% were below 1 year of age, 17.5% were between 1 and 2 years, and 44.5% were over 2 years of age. (This compilation probably included data from major institutions which contributed overlapping data to other surveys and publications.)

Age Versus Stage

The tables showing the relationship between age and clinical stage (another prognostic variable) are based on data from Breslow and McCann (12) and Kinnier-Wilson and Draper (52). Breslow and McCann's (12) statistical estimations of prognosis utilized information on 148 children treated at the Children's Hospital of Philadelphia from 1947 through 1967 and on 112 children studied by the Children's Cancer Study Group A from 1966 to 1968. Kinnier-Wilson and Draper (52) compiled data on 487 cases from cancer registries in Great Britain for children with neuroblastoma from 1962 to 1967. In the latter study, the clinical stage was unknown in 128 patients (26.2%); data were utilized in Table 4 from the remaining 359 patients in whom both stage and age were known. The clinical stage utilized criteria published by Evans et al. (26).

Table 4 shows that 26.8% of the patients were under 1 year of age, 18.5% were between 1 and 2 years, and 54.7% were over 2 years. For the entire patient population, 17.2% were stage I, 13.6% stage II, 9.6% stage III, 48.9% stage IV, and 10.7%

TABLE 4. Stage and age distribution in neuroblastoma

Stage	Ref.	Age (years)			
		Under 1	1 to 2	Over 2	Total
I	52	22	21	40	83
	12	12	4	5	21
		34 (32.7%)[a] (21.0%)[b]	25 (24.0%) (22.3%)	45 (43.3%) (13.6%)	104 (100.0%) (17.2%)
II	52	19	7	21	47
	12	16	7	12	35
		35 (42.7%)[a] (21.6%)[b]	14 (17.1%) (12.5%)	33 (40.2%) (10.0%)	82 (100.0%) (13.6%)
III	52	3	6	22	31
	12	4	8	15	27
		7 (12.1%)[a] (4.3%)[b]	14 (24.1%) (12.5%)	37 (63.8%) (11.2%)	58 (100.0%) (9.6%)
IV	52	21	30	109	160
	12	18	25	93	136
		39 (13.2%)[a] (24.1%)[b]	55 (18.6%) (49.1%)	202 (68.2%) (61.0%)	296 (100.0%) (48.9%)
IV-S	52	28	1	9	38
	12	19	3	5	27
		47 (72.3%)[a] (29.0%)[b]	4 (6.2%) (3.6%)	14 (21.5%) (4.2%)	65 (100.0%) (10.7%)
Total patients		162	112	331	605

[a] Percent of horizontal line total.
[b] Percent of vertical column total.

stage IV-S. The table also provides information on the age parti-
tion (%) for each stage.

Thus, under 1 year of age, 24.1% were stage IV and 29.0%
stage IV-S. In children over 2 years of age, 61% were stage IV
and only 4.2% stage IV-S. Inspection of Table 4 shows that in
the very young (under 1 year of age), there were far more prognostically favorable stages (I and IV-S) and far less prognostically
unfavorable stages (IV) than in children over 2 years of age.

Age Versus Primary Site

A third prognostic variable in neuroblastoma is the site of
the primary lesion. Table 5 examines the relationship between
age and the primary site. (The relationship of clinical stage to
primary site is tabulated in the following section on clinical stage.)

STAGE

The technique for staging neuroblastoma, proposed in 1971
by Evans et al. (26), is now used widely. The criteria for the

TABLE 5. *Relationship of age to primary site in neuroblastoma[a]*

Age (years)	Primary site			All sites
	Abdomen	Thorax	Other	
Under 1	58 (21.7%)[b] (47.9%)[c]	25 (31.2%) (20.7%)	38 (27.1%) (31.4%)	121 (24.8%)
1 to 2	54 (20.2%)[b] (68.4%)[c]	10 (12.5%) (12.7%)	15 (10.7%) (18.9%)	79 (16.2%)
Over 2	155 (58.1%)[b] (54.0%)[c]	45 (56.3%) (15.7%)	87 (62.1%) (30.3%)	287 (58.9%)
All ages	267 (100.0%)[b] (54.8%)[c]	80 (100.0%) (16.4%)	140 (100.0%) (28.7%)	487 (100.0%) (100.0%)

[a] Data from Kinnier-Wilson and Draper (52).
[b] Percent of vertical column total.
[c] Percent of horizontal line total.

various stages are shown in Table 6. The relative frequencies of the various stages among several neuroblastoma populations are indicated in Table 7, which summarizes the data from three reports covering five different series (12,52,101). The relationship of stage to the age of the patient has already been tabulated (Table 4). Information regarding the clinical stage and the site of the primary has been extracted from Zucker's (101) report and is presented in Table 8.

In examining Table 7, some variation in the frequencies of specific stages among the different reports is noticeable. The ranges in the percent frequency of a given stage in the five populations were: stage I, 6.3 to 25.0%; stage II, 4.2 to 14.9%; stage III, 6.4 to 11.9%; stage IV, 32.9 to 56.0%; and stage IV-S, 6.7 to 16.7%.

There are some major implications of these distributions. First, one cannot exclude the probability that the technique and precision of staging vary from one institution to another. Second, in many of the reports, staging was done retrospectively, often years

TABLE 6. *Criteria for staging of childhood neuroblastoma*[a]

Stage	Criteria
I	Tumor confined to the organ or structure of origin.
II	Tumors extending in continuity beyond the organ or structure of origin but not crossing the midline. Regional lymph nodes on the homolateral side may be involved.
III	Tumors extending in continuity beyond the midline. Regional lymph nodes may be involved bilaterally.
IV	Remote disease involving skeleton, organs, soft tissues, or distant lymph node groups.
IV-S	Patients who would otherwise be stage I or II but who have remote disease confined to only one or more of the following sites: liver, skin, or bone marrow (without radiographic evidence of bone metastases on complete skeletal survey).

[a] From Evans et al. (26).

TABLE 7. Stages in neuroblastoma at diagnosis

Stage	Villejuif (101)		Amster-dam (101)		CCSGA[b] (12)		CHOP[c] (12)		Great Britain (52)		Combined total	
	No.	%	No.	%	No.	%	No.	%	No.	%		
I	39	10.0	18	25.0	7	6.3	14	10.4	83	17.0	161	13.5
II	46	11.8	3	4.2	15	13.4	20	14.9	47	9.7	131	11.0
III	37	9.5	5	6.9	11	9.8	16	11.9	31	6.4	100	8.4
IV	197	50.5	32	44.4	61	54.5	75	56.0	160	32.9	525	43.9
IV-S	31	7.9	12	16.7	18	16.1	9	6.7	39	8.0	109	9.1
Unknown	40	10.3	2	2.8	[d]		[d]		127	26.1	169	14.1
	390		72		112		134		487		1,195	

[a]Percent of vertical column total.
[b]CCSGA, Children's Cancer Study Group A.
[c]CHOP, Children's Hospital of Philadelphia.
[d]Numbers of unknown stage not given.

TABLE 8. *Relationship between clinical stage and primary site*[a]

| | Site of primary | | | |
| | Abdomen | | Thorax | |
Stage	No.	%[b]	No.	%
I	12	4.2	22	33.3
II	26	9.0	13	19.7
III	28	9.7	6	9.1
IV	170	59.0	14	21.2
IV-S	27	9.4	1	1.5
Unknown	25	8.7	10	15.2
	288		66	

[a] Data from Zucker (101).
[b] Percent of vertical column total.

after the patient was first seen. This fact, coupled with the difficulty in determining the primary site in some children with disseminated disease, make proper staging impossible. The fraction with unknown stage varied in the reports from 2.8% to as high as 26% of the patients. Third, when survival rates are examined, the magnitude of the overall survival rate can be influenced by the proportions of favorable or unfavorable stages that are present in each neuroblastoma population.

The report by Breslow and McCann (12) includes data from the Philadelphia Children's Hospital and from other members of the Children's Cancer Study Group A. Being the institution and the cooperative group that defined the concept, established the criteria, and field tested the techniques of staging neuroblastoma, their data could be accepted as "standards for comparison" by others deriving similar data.

STAGE IV-S

In 1971, the concept of stage IV-S neuroblastoma was advanced (16,26) to designate those patients "who would otherwise be Stage

I or II, but who have remote disease confined only to one or more of the following sites: liver, skin, or bone marrow." Evidence of skeletal metastases excluded the patient from this category. Clinical experience has demonstrated that patients with IV-S disease have certain additional characteristics. First, most of the patients are babies younger than 13 months. In the initial publication (16), 12 of 16 patients were less than 1 year of age, and 13 of 16 were less than 2 years. In other reports (one of which included the data in the original publication) (12), 72% of 65 IV-S patients were under 1 year of age, and 78% were under 2 years. Compiled data show that among 162 children under 1 year of age, 29% were stage IV-S (see Table 4). Second, children with stage IV-S neuroblastoma have an unexpectedly good prognosis. Evans et al. (26) reported that the overall survival (at 2 years) was 75% of 16 patients. In a larger series, Breslow and McCann (12) calculated the survival rate to be 91% in those under 1 year of age, 54% in those 1 to 2 years, and 42% in those over 2 years. The overall survival was 21/27 (78%). The significance of these survival rates becomes emphasized when it is realized that these children have stage IV disease. Survivals in stage IV patients were 26% for those under 1 year of age and less than 3% in those over 2 years (12).

The importance of considering these patients as a special entity is threefold. First, it has been reported that most of these patients require only minimum treatment (17,24). The danger of overtreatment, with known risk of late effects after such treatment as irradiation, is real. Second, the inclusion of any recognizable group of patients with special prognostic characteristics may interfere with proper interpretation of results of therapy. Third, a careful study of these patients, whose tumors behave unpredictably, may yield meaningful information regarding the biologic nature of neuroblastoma (17,29,78).

While it is difficult to compare the diagnostic precision of one investigator with that of another and even more hazardous to compare two different series of neuroblastoma patients, it may be of interest to at least examine compiled tabulations. As noted on Table 7, the frequencies of stage IV-S patients varied in the five series from 6.7 to 16.7%. The frequency in the compiled data was 9.1% of 1,195 patients. By definition, cases with skeletal metastases are excluded. With additional diagnostic techniques now available, it is possible that lesser involvement of bone can be detected. Although the question of the significance of primitive cells and of tumor cells in bone marrow aspirates of children with neuroblastoma has been examined, the relationship between the presence of tumor cells in the marrow to early skeletal metastasis needs resolution (17,29).

SITE OF PRIMARY TUMOR

The prognostic importance of the site of the primary lesion in neuroblastoma is supported by two types of observations. First, patients with tumors arising in the abdominal area have the poorest prognosis, with those with adrenal primaries faring the worst (19,20,36,52,101). Second, patients with primary tumors arising from the mediastinum appeared to have distinctly better chances for survival (31).

Jaffe (49) has prepared a recent compilation of primary sites of neuroblastoma and corresponding survival rates from 10 reported series. The tumor arose in the thorax in 14% of the cases (with 61% survival), compared to 54% originating in the abdomen (with 20% survival). When the abdominal cases were further subdivided into those of adrenal origin and those of extraadrenal origin, the patients with adrenal origin had the poorest survival (9%) of any primary site category.

In the tabulations prepared for this chapter, the primary sites were divided into abdominal and extraabdominal categories. The abdominal group was subdivided into adrenal and extraadrenal; liver, paravertebral, and retroperitoneal tumors were considered in the abdominal group but pelvic tumors were not. The thoracic (mediastinal) site was considered separately, and cervical primaries were considered under "other."

Table 9 shows the distribution of primary sites from five re-

TABLE 9. *Distribution of primary site of neuroblastoma*

Ref.	No. of patients	Abdominal site (%)			Extraabdominal site (%)		
		Adrenal	Extra-adrenal	Total	Thorax	Other	Total
101	462	18	55	73	16	10	27
52	487	23	36	59	16	25	41
20	173	40	36	77	13	10	23
36	133	50	19	69	8	23	31
19	189	[a]	[a]	71	17	12	29
	1444	27	41	68	15	16	32

[a] Abdominal sites not subdivided.

ported series. The compiled data indicated that 68% of the tumors arose from abdominal sites and 15% within the thorax. Although adrenal and extraadrenal (but abdominal) sites are frequently distinguished in various publications, the difficulty of establishing the organ of origin is indicated by the wide differences among the series for frequency of adrenal primaries, ranging from 18 to 50% of the cases.

With respect to consideration of the relationship of survival to site of primary, other prognostic variables must be examined at the same time. The relationship between age and primary site has already been shown in Table 5. There does not seem to be any significant concentration of older patients among the abdominal cases and no preponderance of younger patients among the thoracic cases. It has been suggested that mediastinal neuroblastomas may not originate from sympathetic ganglia, and hence its biological behavior may be less malignant.

The relationship between primary site and stage was shown in Table 8. It is apparent that patients with abdominal primaries consist of markedly less stage I and significantly more stage IV cases than the patients with thoracic primaries. The difference in the extent of disease (stage) probably accounts for the difference in survival rates between abdominal and thoracic cases.

SURVIVAL STATISTICS

The proper preparation and interpretation of survival statistics must take into consideration the many tumor and patient characteristics that seem to have prognostic significance. Such variables as the age of the patient, the site of the primary lesion, and the extent of the disease (stage) have been discussed in other sections of this chapter. Still other factors that may impact on survival are (a) effectiveness of the treatment, (b) pattern of metastases, (c) histopathologic nature of the tumor, and (d) immunologic status of the patient. Until these variables are identified and the interactions among them clarified, we must utilize tabulations of survival within various categories.

In this section, overall survival is examined first. Data from selected sources then are tabulated to indicate survival separately by age, stage, and site of primary lesion. Finally, at the risk of some repetition, the data have been rearranged to construct tables that relate survival to other factors, specifically, survival by age and stage, survival by age and site of primary tumor, and survival by stage and primary site.

Overall Survival

While the calculation of a single overall survival rate for a given series, including all patients, may be crude and oversimplified, such figures permit a perspective over time and across therapeutic epochs. It is reasonable to assume that significant improvements in the results of treatment would be reflected by an improvement in survival rate. As a corollary, the failure to discern any change in survival rate could be interpreted as the result of ineffective treatment. Table 10 shows some of the reported survival experiences, each over a relatively short period of time.

Although neuroblastoma may be one of the relatively common solid tumors of childhood, it is still numerically rare. It is difficult for any single institution to accumulate meaningful numbers of

TABLE 10. *Overall survival rates in neuroblastoma*

Ref.	Time period	Stages	No. of patients	Percent survival
92	1956	All	84	23[a]
92	1962	All	142	22[a]
92	1956	III–IV	41	13[a]
92	1962	III–IV	96	22[a]
64	1966–1968	III–IV	70	13[a]
52	1962–1967	All	487	23.4
12	1966–1967	All	142	31.3

[a] Extrapolated from survival curves.

cases within a short time span. All available data that meet the time restriction and volume requirement are multiinstitutional and compiled. There is an obvious need to obtain more recent survival data to assess current therapeutic performance.

One randomized investigation by the Children's Cancer Study Group A examined the effectiveness of cyclophosphamide adjuvant chemotherapy in nonmetastatic neuroblastoma (stages I, II, and III) patients (21). No difference was found either in duration of disease-free survival or in survival rate between those who received chemotherapy and those who did not.

Age and Survival

Practically all sizable series of patients indicate that the young age groups have the best survival. Some recent publications have been compiled in Table 11 to illustrate this.

Stage and Survival

The general trend for survival rates to decrease as the extent of the disease (stage) increases is shown in Table 12. The good prognosis in stage IV-S disease is apparent.

TABLE 11. *Survival (2 years +) in relation to age in neuroblastoma (all stages, all sites)*

Age (years)	Breslow and McCann (12)		Kinnier-Wilson and Draper (52)		Zucker (101)	
	No.	%	No.	%	No.	%
Under 1	51/69	73.9	59/121	48.8	77/110	70.0
1 to 2	12/47	25.5	19/79	24.1	48/235[a]	20.4
Over 2	16/130	12.3	36/287	12.5		
All ages	79/246	32.1	114/487	23.4	125/345	36.2

[a] Includes all children older than 1 year of age.

Site and Survival

Compiled data show that patients with the primary tumor arising in the thorax have better survival rates (Table 13).

Age/Stage and Survival

Breslow and McCann (12) have provided analyses that permit estimation of survival probabilities based on age and stage (Table 14).

TABLE 12. *Stage and survival rate in neuroblastoma (all ages, all sites)*

Stage	Survival rate (%)		
	Breslow and McCann (12)	Zucker (101)	Kinnier-Wilson and Draper (52)
I	85.7	94.9	59.0
II	62.9	73.3	46.8
III	37.0	51.4	19.4
IV	5.9	9.3	5.0
IV-S	77.8	60.0	48.7

TABLE 13. *Primary site and survival rate in neuroblastoma (all ages, all stages)*

Primary site	Survival rate (%)	
	Kinnier-Wilson and Draper (52)	Zucker (101)
Abdomen	14.6	27
Adrenal	10.7	
Extraadrenal	21.8	
Thorax	41.3	75
Other	25.6	

Age/Primary Site and Survival

Data from Kinnier-Wilson and Draper (52) have been extracted for Table 15 to examine how age and primary site relate to survival. Evans et al. (22) have analyzed the relationships among site, stage, age, and survival. They found that tumors originating above the diaphragm had better survival than those below, but the difference was not statistically significant. Additionally, they did not find age to be significantly related to primary sites above or below the diaphragm.

TABLE 14. *Percent survival by age and stage in neuroblastoma[a]*

Age (years)	Stage				
	I	II	III	IV	IV-S
Under 1	97	89	82	26	91
1 to 2	77	49	36	4	54
Over 2	67	37	26	3	42

[a] Data published by Breslow and McCann (12).

TABLE 15. *Percent survival by age and primary site in neuroblastoma (all stages)[a]*

Site of primary	Age (years)		
	Under 1	1 to 2	Over 2
Abdomen	41.1	14.8	7.5
Adrenal	16.7	12.9	5.9
Extraadrenal	58.1	17.3	8.3
Thorax	68.0	70.0	20.0
Other	52.1	26.7	18.1

[a] Data compiled from Kinnier-Wilson and Draper (52).

CHEMOTHERAPY

The data do not yet indicate a consistently significant improvement in the survival rate as the result of chemotherapy during the past two or three decades. However, temporary responses (often of striking degree) have occurred in metastatic disease after the administration of a number of drugs. Table 16 lists many of the drugs that have been and are being used in various chemotherapeutic regimens. Although current programs generally utilize the drugs in various combinations, the table provides a brief assessment of reported results from single agent therapy as well as from combination treatment.

The data have been tabulated from studies (phase II) on disseminated neuroblastoma (stage IV). Stage IV disease constitutes the majority of neuroblastoma cases, and responses can be evaluated objectively. On the other hand, interpretation of the results must include the probability that in most phase II investigations, the patients will have had prior therapy, often very intensive, with the agents considered to be the most effective. Also, in tabulations of this type, the designation of "response" is imprecise. The term includes "complete" as well as "partial" regressions,

TABLE 16. *Chemotherapy in neuroblastoma*

Drug(s)	Refs.	Response rate	Comments
Cyclophosphamide	21,34,53, 66,86,93, 97	Up to 60–70%	This alkylating agent has consistently produced responses of varying degrees and durations in metastatic neuroblastoma. It is a key drug in most combination regimens. A higher rate of responses seems to occur when given on a high dose intermittent schedule (34). No demonstrable effect on survival was noted in stage I, II, and III cases when used as adjuvant chemotherapy in a randomized study (21).
VCR	50,66,84, 87,90	30–40%	Used singly, VCR also produces temporary regression of metastatic disease in moderate numbers. Because of lack of overlapping toxicity with most other drugs, it is frequently used in combination regimens.
Cyclophosphamide plus VCR	28,51,76, 81,86,87	40–80%	This widely used combination produces regression of metastatic nodules. Complete although temporary responses can be seen in about 25%. The response rate remains the same whether the two drugs are given concurrently, sequentially, or alternately (81).
Daunomycin	23,80,91 96	10–35%	Somewhat conflicting reports have been published about the effectiveness of daunomycin in neuroblastoma. At best, the results suggest that the drug should be used in combination with other drugs.
Adriamycin	23,77,95	20–40%	Compiled results indicate a somewhat higher activity against neuroblastoma than daunomycin. This drug probably should be combined with other drugs.
VCR plus cyclophosphamide plus daunomycin	46	50%	This reasonable combination has not significantly improved the results of two-drug combination of VCR and cyclophosphamide.
VCR plus cyclophosphamide plus adriamycin	37	50%	Another reasonable combination of partially effective drugs but summation of activities has not resulted.

Regimen	Reference	Response	Comments
DTIC	33	15%	Used singly, DTIC has some but not impressive activity. It is used generally in combination with adriamycin.
DTIC plus adriamycin	14,63	10–35%	Published results so far do not indicate greater antitumor activity from the combination than from adriamycin alone.
cis-Platinum (DDP)	65,72,75	15–35%	Although risk of toxicity is significant, moderate antitumor activity has been noted in advanced disease after use of DDP.
Peptichemio	18,73	80%	European studies have reported some early encouraging results with this new drug (a mixture of six synthetic peptides of m-L-phenylalanine mustard). The drug has alkylating action and considerable toxicity.
VM-26	79	20%	This semisynthetic derivative of podophyllotoxin used singly has only slight antitumor activity but apparently a good effect on bone marrow metastases.
HN₂ plus VCR plus adria-mycin	49		Nitrogen mustard (HN₂) may still be useful in combination regimens. This particular program is used as adjuvant therapy for stages I and II disease.
HN₂ plus VCR plus adria-mycin plus DTIC	49	75%	Good responses have been reported in stages III and IV disease
VCR plus cyclophos-phamide plus F3TDR plus papaverine	43,45,71	50–80%	This regimen combines cytotoxic agents and "maturation-inducing" agents. Although toxicity is prominent, responses in far advanced neuroblastoma have been reported.
VCR plus cyclophos-phamide plus adriamy-cin plus actinomycin D	44		Another multiagent combination, but no improvement in results over VCR-cyclophosphamide-daunomycin combination was noted.
VCR plus cyclophos-phamide plus DTIC	32,35,39	65%	Early results seem promising.
VCR plus cyclophos-phamide plus adriamy-cin plus 5-FU	13	65%	In multidrug combinations, it is difficult to sort out the responses to individual drugs, e.g., the contribution of 5-FU.

and the durations of the responses vary. Thus the rates provide only an approximate estimation of the antitumor activities.

A representative but not comprehensive selection of published references is given.

REFERENCES

1. American Academy of Pediatrics (1968): *J. Pediatr. Surg.,* 3:191–193.
2. Beckwith, J. B., and Martin, R. F. (1968): Observations on the histopathology of neuroblastomas. *J. Pediatr. Surg.,* 3:106–110.
3. Beckwith, J. B., and Perrin, E. V. (1963): In situ neuroblastomas: A contribution to the natural history of neural crest tumors. *Am. J. Pathol.,* 43:1089–1104.
4. Bernstein, I., Hellström, I., Hellström, K. E., and Wright, P. W. (1976): Immunity to tumor antigens: Potential implications in human neuroblastoma. *J. Natl. Cancer Inst.,* 57:711–715.
5. Bill, A. H. (1969): The implications of immune reactions to neuroblastoma. *Surgery,* 66:415–418.
6. Bill, A. H. (1971): Immune aspects of neuroblastoma. Current information. *Am. J. Surg.,* 122:142–147.
7. Bill, A. H., Jr., Koop, C. E., and Johnson, D. G. (1968): Conference on The Biology of Neuroblastoma. *J. Pediatr. Surg.,* 3:103–193.
8. Bill, A. H., Seibert, E. S., Beckwith, J. B., and Hartmann, J. R. (1969): Nerve growth factor and nerve growth-stimulating activity in sera from normal and neuroblastoma patients. *J. Natl. Cancer Inst.,* 43:1221–1230.
9. Bohuon, C. (editor) (1966): Neuroblastomas: Biochemical studies. *Recent Results Cancer Res.,* 2:1–72.
10. Bolande, R. P. (1971): Benignity of neonatal tumors and concept of cancer repression in early life. *Am. J. Dis. Child.,* 122:12–14.
11. Bradshaw, R. A. (1978): Nerve growth factor. *Annu. Rev. Biochem.,* 47:191–216.
12. Breslow, N., and McCann, B. (1971): Statistical estimation of prognosis for children with neuroblastoma. *Cancer Res.,* 31:2098–2103.
13. Cangir, A., Falletta, J. M., Ragab, A. H., and McMillan, C. (1978): Combination chemotherapy with adriamycin, cyclophosphamide, vincristine, and 5-fluorouracil (AD-CON-FU) in children with metastatic solid tumors and untreated rare tumors. *Proc. AACR ASCO,* 19:391 (Abstr.).
14. Cangir, A., Morgan, S. K., Land, V. J., Pullen, J., Starling, K. A., and Nitschke, R. (1976): Combination chemotherapy with adriamycin and dimethyl triazeno imidazole carboxamide in children with metastatic solid tumors. *Med. Pediatr. Oncol.,* 2:183–190.
15. Cole, W. H. (1976): Spontaneous regression of cancer and the importance of finding its cause. *Natl. Cancer Inst. Monogr.,* 44:5–9.
16. D'Angio, G. J., Evans, A. E., and Koop, C. E. (1971): Special pattern of widespread neuroblastoma with a favourable prognosis. *Lancet,* 1:1046.

17. D'Angio, G. J., Lyser, K. M., and Urunay, G. (1971): Neuroblastoma, Stage IV-S: A special entity? *Clin. Bull.,* 1:61–65.
18. DeBernardi, B., Comelli, A., Cozzuto, C., Lamedica, G., Mori, P. G., and Massino, L. (1978): Peptichemio in advanced neuroblastoma. *Cancer Treat. Rep.,* 62:811–817.
19. de Lorimier, A. A., Bragg, K. U., and Linden, G. (1969): Neuroblastoma in childhood. *Am. J. Dis. Child.,* 118:441–450.
20. Duckett, J. W., and Koop, C. E. (1977): Neuroblastoma. *Urol. Clin. North Am.,* 4:285–295.
21. Evans, A. E., Albo, V., D'Angio, G. J., Finklestein, J. Z., Leiken, S., Santulli, T., Weiner, J., and Hammond, G. D. (1976): Cyclophosphamide treatment of patients with localized and regional neuroblastoma. A randomized study. *Cancer,* 38:655–660.
22. Evans, A. E., Albo, V., D'Angio, G. J., Finklestein, J. Z., Leiken, S., Santulli, T., Weiner, J., and Hammond, G. D. (1976): Factors influencing survival of children with nonmetastatic neuroblastoma. *Cancer,* 38:661–666.
23. Evans, A. E., Baehner, R. L., Chard, R. L., Jr., Leikin, S. L., Pang, E. M., and Pierce, M. (1974): Comparison of daunorubicin with adriamycin in the treatment of late-stage childhood solid tumors. *Cancer Chemother. Rep.,* 58:671–676.
24. Evans, A. E., Chard, R., and Baum, E. (1978): Do children with IV-S neuroblastoma require treatment? *Proc. AACR ASCO,* 19:367 (Abstr.).
25. Evans, A. E., D'Angio, G. J., and Koop, C. E. (1976): Diagnosis and treatment of neuroblastoma. *Pediatr. Clin. North Am.,* 23:161–170.
26. Evans, A. E., D'Angio, G. J., and Randolph, J. (1971): A proposed staging for children with neuroblastoma. Children's Cancer Study Group A. *Cancer,* 27:374–378.
27. Evans, A. E., Gerson, J., and Schnaufer, L. (1976): Spontaneous regression of neuroblastoma. *Natl. Cancer Inst. Monogr.,* 44:49–54.
28. Evans, A. E., Heyn, R. M., Newton, W. A., Jr., and Leikin, S. L. (1969): Vincristine sulfate and cyclophosphamide for children with metastatic neuroblastoma. *JAMA,* 207:1325–1327.
29. Evans, A. E., and Hummeler, K. (1973): The significance of primitive cells in marrow aspirates of children with neuroblastoma. *Cancer,* 32:906–912.
30. Everson, T. C. (1964): Spontaneous regression of cancer. *Ann. NY Acad. Sci.,* 114:721–735.
31. Filler, R. M., Traggis, D. G., Jaffe, N., and Vawter, G. F. (1972): Favorable outlook for children with mediastinal neuroblastoma. *J. Pediatr. Surg.,* 7:136–143.
32. Finklestein, J. Z. (1976): Neuroblastoma: A unique solid tumor of childhood. In: *Trends in Childhood Cancer,* edited by M. H. Donaldson and H. G. Seydel, pp. 107–121. Wiley, New York.
33. Finkelstein, J. Z., Albo, V., Ertel, I., and Hammond, D. (1975): 5-(3,3-Dimethyl-1-triazeno) imidazole-4-carboxamide in the treatment of solid tumors in children. *Cancer Chemother. Rep.,* 59:351–357.

34. Finkelstein, J. Z., Hittle, R. E., and Hammond, G. D. (1969): Evaluation of a high dose cyclophosphamide regimen in childhood tumors. *Cancer,* 23:1239–1242.
35. Finklestein, J. Z., Leikin, S., Evans, A., Klemperer, M., Bernstein, I., Hittle, R., and Hammond, G. D. (1974): Combination chemotherapy for metastatic neuroblastoma. *Proc. AACR ASCO,* 15:44 (Abstr.).
36. Fortner, J., Nicastri, A., and Murphy, M. L. (1968): Neuroblastoma: Natural history and results of treating 133 cases. *Ann. Surg.,* 167:132–142.
37. Gasparini, M., Bellani, F. F., Musumeci, R., and Bonadonna, G. (1974): Response and survival of patients with metastatic neuroblastoma after combination chemotherapy with adriamycin, cyclophosphamide, and vincristine. *Cancer Chemother. Rep.,* 58:365–370.
38. Gerson, J. M., and Koop, C. E. (1974): Neuroblastoma. *Semin. Oncol.,* 1:35–46.
39. Grosfeld, J. L., Schatzlein, M., Ballantine, T. V. N., Weetman, R. M., and Baehner, R. L. (1978): Metastatic neuroblastoma: Factors influencing survival. *J. Pediatr. Surg.,* 13:59–65.
40. Gitlow, S. E., Dziedzic, B., Strauss, L., Greenwood, S. M., and Dziedzic, S. W. (1973): Biochemical and histologic determinants in the prognosis of neuroblastoma. *Cancer,* 32:898–905.
41. Gross, R. E., Farber, S., and Martin, L. W. (1959): Neuroblastoma sympatheticum. A study and report of 217 cases. *Pediatrics,* 23:1179–1191.
42. Hellström, K. E., and Hellström, I. (1972): Immunity to neuroblastomas and melanomas. *Annu. Rev. Med.,* 23:19–38.
43. Helson, L. (1975): Management of disseminated neuroblastoma. *CA,* 25:264–277.
44. Helson, L., and Denoix, L. (1973): Four drug sequential chemotherapy for metastatic neuroblastoma. *Eur. J. Cancer,* 9:883–885.
45. Helson, L., Helson, C., Peterson, R. F., and Das, S. K. (1976): A rationale for the treatment of metastatic neuroblastoma. *J. Natl. Cancer Inst.,* 57:727–729.
46. Helson, L., Vanichayangkul, P., Tan, C. T., Wollner, N., and Murphy, M. L. (1972): Combination intermittent chemotherapy for patients with disseminated neuroblastoma. *Cancer Chemother. Rep.,* 56:499–503.
47. Horn, R. C., Jr., Koop, C. E., and Kiesewetter, W. B. (1956): Neuroblastoma in childhood. Clinicopathologic study of forty-four cases. *Lab. Invest.,* 5:106–119.
48. Hughes, M., Marsden, H. B., and Palmer, M. K. (1974): Histologic patterns of neuroblastoma related to prognosis and clinical staging. *Cancer,* 34:1706–1711.
49. Jaffe, N. (1976): Neuroblastoma: Review of the literature and an examination of factors contributing to its enigmatic character. *Cancer Treat. Rev.,* 3:61–82.
50. James, D. H., Jr., and George, P. (1964): Vincristine in children with malignant solid tumors. *J. Pediatr.,* 64:534–541.
51. James, D. H., Jr., Hustu, O., Wrenn, E. L., Jr., and Pinkel, D. (1965):

Combined chemotherapy of childhood neuroblastoma. *JAMA,* 194:123–126.

52. Kinnier-Wilson, L. M., and Draper, G. J. (1974): Neuroblastoma, its natural history and prognosis: A study of 487 cases. *Br. Med. J.,* 3:301–307.
53. Kontras, S. B., and Newton, W. A., Jr. (1961): Cyclophosphamide (cytoxan) therapy of childhood neuroblastoma. Preliminary report. *Cancer Chemother. Rep.,* 12:39–50.
54. Koop, C. E. (1968): Neuroblastoma: Two year survival and treatment correlations. *J. Pediatr. Surg.,* 3:178–179.
55. Koop, C. E. (1971): Factors affecting survival in neuroblastoma. *J. Pediatr. Surg.,* 3:113–114.
56. Koop, C. E. (1972): The neuroblastoma. *Prog. Pediatr. Surg.,* 3:1–28.
57. Koop, C. E., and Johnson, D. G. (1971): Neuroblastoma: An assessment of therapy in reference to staging. *J. Pediatr. Surg.,* 6:595–600.
58. Koop, C. E., and Schnaufer, L. (1975): The management of abdominal neuroblastoma. *Cancer,* 35:905–909.
59. Kumar, S., Steward, J. K., Waghe, M., Pearson, D., Edwards, D. C., Fenton, E. L., and Griffith, A. H. (1970): The administration of the nerve growth factor to children with widespread neuroblastoma. *J. Pediatr. Surg.,* 5:18–22.
60. LaBrosse, E. H., Comoy, E., Bohuon, C., Zucker, J-M., and Schweisguth, O. (1975): Catecholamine metabolism in neuroblastoma. *J. Natl. Cancer Inst.,* 57:633–638.
61. Lauder, I., and Aherne, W. (1972): The significance of lymphocytic infiltration in neuroblastoma. *Br. J. Cancer,* 26:321–330.
62. Laug, W. E., Siegel, S. E., Shaw, K. N. F., Landing, B., Baptista, J., and Gutenstein, M. (1978): Initial urinary catecholamine metabolite concentrations and prognosis in neuroblastoma. *Pediatrics,* 62:77–83.
63. Leikin, S., Bernstein, I., Evans, A., Finklestein, J., Hittle, R., and Klemperer, M. (1978): Use of combination adriamycin and DTIC in children with advanced Stage IV neuroblastoma. *Cancer Chemother. Rep.,* 59:1015–1018.
64. Leikin, S., Evans, A., Heyn, R., and Newton, W. (1974): The impact of chemotherapy on advanced neuroblastoma. Survival of patients diagnosed in 1956, 1962, and 1966–68 in Children's Cancer Study Group A. *J. Pediatr.,* 84:131–134.
65. Leventhal, B. G., and Freeman, A. (1979): Cis-diammine dichloro platinum. A Phase II study in pediatric malignancies. *Proc. AACR ASCO,* 20:197 (Abstr.).
66. Livingston, R. B., and Carter, S. K. (1970): *Single Agents In Cancer Chemotherapy* Plenum, New York.
67. Marsden, H. B., and Steward, J. K. (1976): Tumors of the sympathetic system. *Recent Results Cancer Res.,* 13:194–244.
68. Martin, R. F., and Beckwith, J. B. (1968): Lymphoid infiltrates in neuroblastomas: Their occurrence and prognostic significance. *J. Pediatr. Surg.,* 3:161–164.

69. Mobley, W. C., Server, A. C., Ishii, D. N., Riopelle, R. J., and Shooter, E. M. (1978): Nerve growth factor. *N. Engl. J. Med.,* 297:1096–1104, 1149–1158, 1211–1218.

70. Necheles, T. F., Rausen, A. R., Kung, F. H., and Pochedly, C. (1978): Immunochemotherapy in advanced neuroblastoma. *Cancer,* 41:1282–1288.

71. Nitschke, R., Cangir, A., Crist, W., and Berry, D. H. (1979): Intensive chemotherapy for metastatic neuroblastoma. *Proc. AACR ASCO,* 20:392 (Abstr.).

72. Nitschke, R., Starling, K. A., Vats, T., and Bryan, H. (1978): Cis-diamminedichloroplatinum in childhood malignancies. *Med. Pediatr. Oncol.,* 4:127–132.

73. Otten, J., and Maurus, R. (1978): Clinical trial of peptichemio in solid tumors of childhood. *Cancer Treat. Rep.,* 62:1015–1019.

74. Pochedly, C. (editor) (1976): *Neuroblastoma.* Publishing Sciences Group, Acton, Massachusetts.

75. Pratt, C. B., Hayes, F. A., Green, A. A., Evans, W. E., Senzer, N., Howarth, C., and Ransom, J. L. (1979): Phase II—pharmacokinetic study of cis-platinum diamminedichloride (CPDD) in children with solid tumors. *Proc. AACR ASCO,* 20:361 (Abstr.).

76. Pratt, C. B., James, D. H., Jr., Holton, C. P., and Pinkel, D. (1965): Combination therapy including vincristine for malignant solid tumors in children. *Cancer Chemother. Rep.,* 52:489–495.

77. Ragab, A. H., Sutow, W. W., Komp, D. M., Starling, K. A., Lyon, G. M., Jr., and George, S. (1975): Adriamycin in the treatment of childhood solid tumors. *Cancer,* 36:1572–1576.

78. Rangecroft, L., Lauder, I., and Wagget, J. (1978): Spontaneous maturation of Stage IV-S neuroblastoma. *Arch. Dis. Child.,* 53:815–817.

79. Rivera, G., Green, A., Hayes, A., Avery, T., Pratt, C. (1977): Epipodophyllotoxin VM-26 in the treatment of childhood neuroblastoma. *Cancer Treat. Rep.,* 61:1243–1248.

80. Samuels, L. D., Newton, W. A., Jr., and Heyn, R. (1971): Daunorubicin therapy in advanced neuroblastoma. *Cancer,* 27:831–834.

81. Sawitsky, A. (1970): Vincristine and cyclophosphamide therapy in generalized neuroblastoma. A collaborative study. *Am. J. Dis. Child.,* 119:308–313.

82. Schwartz, A. D., Dadash-Zadeh, M., Lee, H., and Swaney, J.J. (1974): Spontaneous regression of disseminated neuroblastoma. *J. Pediatr.,* 85:760–763.

83. Schweisguth, O. (1968): Treatment of neuroblastoma. *J. Pediatr. Surg.,* 3:183–184.

84. Selawry, O., Holland, J. F., and Wolman, I. J. (1968): Effect of vincristine on malignant solid tumors in children. *Cancer Chemother. Rep.,* 52:497–500.

85. Societé Internationale d'Oncologie Pédiatriqué (1974): Proceedings of conference on neuroblastoma. *Maandschr. Kindergeneesk.,* 42:369–490.

86. Starling, K. A., Sutow, W. W., Donaldson, M. H., Land, V. J., and Lane,

D. M. (1974): Drug trials in neuroblastoma: Cyclophosphamide alone; vincristine plus cyclophosphamide; 6-mercaptopurine plus 6-methylmercaptopurine riboside; and cytosine arabinoside alone. *Cancer Chemother. Rep.,* 58:683–688.

87. Sullivan, M. P., Nora, A. H., Kulapongs, P., Lane, D. M., Windmiller, J., and Thurman, W. G. (1969): Evaluation of vincristine sulfate and cyclophosphamide chemotherapy for metastatic neuroblastoma. *Pediatrics,* 44:685–694.

88. Sutow, W. W. (1958): Prognosis in neuroblastoma of childhood. *AMA J. Dis. Child.,* 96:299–305.

89. Sutow, W. W. (1968): Chemotherapeutic considerations in neuroblastoma. *J. Pediatr. Surg.,* 3:132–134.

90. Sutow, W. W., (1968): Vincristine therapy for malignant solid tumors in children (except Wilms' tumor). *Cancer Chemother. Rep.,* 52:485–487.

91. Sutow, W. W., Fernbach, D. J., Thurman, W. G., Holton, C. P., and Watkins, W. L. (1970): Daunomycin in the treatment of metastatic neuroblastoma. *Cancer Chemother. Rep.,* 54:283–290.

92. Sutow, W. W., Gehan, E. A., Heyn, R. M., Kung, F. H., Miller, R. W., Murphy, M. L., and Traggis, D. G. (1970): Comparison of survival curves, 1956 versus 1962, in children with Wilms' tumor and neuroblastoma. *Pediatrics,* 45:800–811.

93. Sweeney, M. J., Tuttle, A. H., Etteldorf, J. N., and Whittington, G. L. (1962): Cyclophosphamide in the treatment of common neoplastic diseases of childhood. *J. Pediatr.,* 61:702–708.

94. Symposium on Advances in Neuroblastoma Research (1976): *J. Natl. Cancer Inst.,* 57:613–735.

95. Tan, C., Rosen, G., Ghavimi, F., Haghbin, M., Helson, L., Wollner, N., and Murphy, M. L. (1975): Adriamycin in pediatric malignancies. *Cancer Chemother. Rep.,* 6(3):259–266.

96. Tan, C., Tasaka, H., Yu, K-P., Murphy, M. L., and Karnofsky, D. A. (1967): Daunomycin, an antitumor antibiotic, in the treatment of neoplastic disease. *Cancer,* 20:333–353.

97. Thurman, W. G., Fernbach, D. J., and Sullivan, M. P. (1964): Cyclophosphamide therapy in childhood neuroblastoma. *N. Engl. J. Med.,* 270:1336–1340.

98. Voorhess, M. L., and Gardner, L. I. (1961): Urinary excretion of norepinephrine, epinephrine, and 3-methoxy-4-hydroxymandelic acid by children with neuroblastoma. *J. Clin. Endocrinol. Metab.,* 21:321–335.

99. Young, J. L., Jr., Heise, H. W., Silverberg, E., and Myers, M. H. (1978): Cancer incidence, survival and mortality for children under 15 years of age. *Am. Cancer Soc.,* 16 pp.

100. Young, J. L., Jr., and Miller, R. W. (1975): Incidence of malignant tumors in U.S. children. *J. Pediatr.,* 86:254–258.

101. Zucker, J. M. (1974): Retrospective study of 462 neuroblastomas treated between 1950 and 1970. *Maandschr. Kindergeneesk.,* 42:369–385.

6

Wilms' Tumor

Comprehensive reviews (46,55,56,59), analyses of institutional (28) and regional (22,27) experiences, and reports from large-scale cooperative studies (8,29,38) have recently documented the clinical characteristics of and therapeutic results in Wilms' tumor. Except for a brief tabulation of clinical parameters, this chapter does not attempt still another compiled summary of the published reports. Rather, the purposes are to identify specific clinical areas where significant progress has been made in the past decade and to assess the therapeutic attitudes currently being maintained.

The major clinical investigations are now targeted on four important aspects: (a) identification of prognostic factors and utilization of the factors as determinants of therapy, (b) refinement of treatment regimens to obtain maximum results with minimum morbidity, (c) evaluation of the quality of long-term survival, and (d) efforts through genetic and epidemiologic investigations to define the population at risk of developing Wilms' tumor (31,51).

CLINICAL PARAMETERS

Incidence

Current estimates of the frequency of Wilms' tumor in the childhood population within the United States are shown in Table 1. Direct comparison of these two estimates of incidence must consider the difference in geographic coverage between these two studies (65).

Based on international epidemiologic statistics and on data from a special study by the International Union Against Cancer,

TABLE 1. *Incidence of Wilms' tumor in children under 15 years of age*

Ref.	Period of study	White		Black	
		Percent of total cancer	Rate per 1,000,000 population	Percent of total cancer	Rate per 1,000,000 population
SEER program[a] (65)	1973–1976	5.7	6.9	8.1	7.6
Third National Cancer Survey (66)	1969–1971	6.1	7.5	8.0	7.8

[a] Surveillance, Epidemiology and End Results Program, National Cancer Institute.

it has been proposed that Wilms' tumor occurs throughout the world with a remarkably stable, constant incidence (12,20). The incidence does not appear to be affected by race, climate, or environment. For these reasons, Wilms' tumor has been suggested as an index reference cancer for studies of human cancer incidence.

Age and Sex Distribution

Compiled data from several recent publications have been tabulated to obtain a breakdown of the occurrence of Wilms' tumor with respect to age (Table 2). In these tabulations, the median age was slightly under 3 years. About 15% of the patients were infants less than 12 months of age. The peak incidence for Wilms' tumor occurred between 1 and 3 years of age, accounting for 38% of all cases. An analysis of 1,185 cases reported in several large series indicated that 51% of the patients were male and 49% female (55).

TABLE 2. *Age distribution of Wilms' tumor among 974 reported cases*[a]

Age (years)	No. of patients	Percent of total	Cumulative (%)
Under 1	143	14.7	14.7
1–2	191	19.6	34.3
2–3	176	18.1	52.4
3–4	148	15.2	67.6
4–5	102	10.5	78.1
5–6	80	8.2	86.3
6–7	54	5.5	91.8
7–8	25	2.6	94.4
Over 8	55	5.6	100.0
	974	100.0	

[a] Adapted from Sutow (55) and including data from Silva-Sosa and Gonzalez-Cerva (48).

TABLE 3. *Anomalies in 547 Wilms' tumor patients*[a]

Anomaly	No.	Incidence (%)
Hemihypertrophy	16	2.9
Aniridia	6	1.1
G-U tract	24	4.4
Other anomalies		
Other musculoskeletal anomalies	16	2.9
Other eye anomalies	5	0.9
Hamartoma	43	7.9
Miscellaneous	7	1.3

[a] From Pendergrass (44) (NWTS-1).

Associated Congenital Anomalies

Data accumulated in the conduct of cooperative clinical trials now permit a more precise quantitation of the increased frequency of aniridia, hemihypertrophy, and other congenital malformations in patients with Wilms' tumor (16,39–41). Pendergrass (44) has analyzed the flow sheet information on 547 patients registered on the first National Wilms' Tumor Study (NWTS-1) (Table 3).

The possible etiologic significance of these associations have been discussed in several publications (31,50,51). Of equal importance are the genetic implications of the associations as potential "markers" to identify the hereditary cases of Wilms' tumor and the population at greatest risk for developing the tumor (50,52).

PROGNOSTIC FACTORS

With the initiation of randomized cooperative studies (8,29, 38,43), large amounts of controlled data are being generated in a relatively short period of time from a great number of patients under treatment using protocol defined guidelines. Analyses of these data now permit recognition of prognostic variables and better documentation of the clinical behavior of the tumor under treatment (5,10,43). Among the major factors that predict for relapse and for mortality are anaplastic or sarcomatous histology, specimen weight over 250 g, and positive regional lymph nodes. Type of chemotherapy and age over 2 years seem to be associated with disease-free survival but not with mortality (5). Such factors as laterality, capsular penetration, intrarenal vascular invasion, direct regional extension, and operative spillage have lesser effects (5).

By defining the patient population at the greatest relative risk of treatment failure, the prognostic factors can be utilized as significant determinants of the nature and intensity of treatment programs.

Group

The extent of the disease at diagnosis and the degree to which the tumor could be surgically excised have been utilized in the NWTS to determine the clinical group or stage of the disease in the patient (7). This assessment is based on clinical diagnostic findings, surgeon's evaluation at the operating table, and pathologist's confirmation. At present, this NWTS schema has been utilized in the major prospective studies of Wilms' tumor.

Five groups (stages) are defined on the basis of criteria as shown: group I, tumor limited to kidney and completely resected; group II, tumor extends beyond kidney but is completely resected; group III, residual nonhematogenous tumor confined to abdomen; group IV, hematogenous metastases; and group V, bilateral renal involvement.

Results from the cooperative data study indicated, as was anticipated, that survival decreased as the magnitude of the disease (group) increased. In NWTS, the differences in survival may have been even greater among the different groups had the treatment been constant for all groups (Table 4). In NWTS, more intensive therapy was utilized in those groups considered to represent more extensive disease.

TABLE 4. *Grouping/staging versus prognosis*

| Study[a] | Group (stage) | No. of patients | Actuarial survival at 3 years (%) | |
			Disease-free	Overall
MRC-AMD (38)	I	23	73	86
	II	17	41	52
	III	15	40	59
MRC-VCR (38)	I	22	91	100
	II	17	71	76
	III	14	62	69
SIOP (29)	I	58	49	92
	II	84	62	84
	III	53	44	76
NWTS-1 [b] (8)	I (regimen A)	77	83	97
	I (regimen B)	77	71	92
	II and III (regimen C)	59	81	86

[a] In these studies, infants under 1 year of age were excluded. Chemotherapy remained constant irrespective of grouping for each treatment study regimen. The SIOP clinical trials investigated two schedules of AMD without regard to grouping. MRC, Medical Research Council; SIOP, International Society of Pediatric Oncology.

[b] In NWTS, the treatments varied with clinical group. Results from groups II and III were combined for the analysis, and data for regimen C only (best survival) were included in the table.

Treatment

The impact of multimodal and intensive therapy programs on survival in the past is indicated by progressively improving cure rates noted on historic reviews (treatment before 1970) (Table 5) as well as by analysis of data from recent statistically controlled prospective studies (Table 4).

Based on past and recent results, the current therapeutic concepts can be summarized as follows:

1. In the past, two chemotherapeutic agents, actinomycin D (AMD) (15,63) and vincristine (VCR) (54,61) were shown to

TABLE 5. *Reported cure rates in Wilms' tumor*[a]

Treatment	No. of cases	No. of cures	Percent cures
Surgery alone	1,018	192	19
Surgery plus radiotherapy	2,449	753	31
Surgery + radiotherapy + AMD	301	195	65

[a]Only data from American and Canadian sources (55) treated before 1970. These data are of historic interest but do not permit detailed analysis since no prospective grouping/staging system was utilized.

have significant antitumor activity against Wilms' tumor. The potentiation of X-ray effects by AMD was reported from early studies (8,9). More recently, adriamycin (ADR) also was meaningful, effective against metastatic Wilms' tumor (2). The results from collaborative studies indicate that two- and three-drug combinations are more effective than single agent chemotherapy (8,10,43).

2. Improvement in survival resulted from improvement in treatment techniques, primarily from multimodal approaches and more effective utilization of chemotherapy regimens.

3. Analysis of treatment results must take into account the existence of other prognostic factors. Among the most important of these are the extent of the disease in the patient (group/stage) and the histopathologic characteristics of the tumor. Translated into practical considerations, the milieu of interacting factors influences the selection of the therapeutic approach and the evaluation of the therapeutic result.

4. The prognostically worse group of patients needs the most intensive treatment. This group includes primarily those with tumors that are histopathologically unfavorable and those with extensive disease (groups III and IV).

5. Even among prognostically favorable patients, treatment failures occur in varying numbers. Efforts must continue to identify the potential failures, and treatment must be intensified once the patients at risk are known.

6. When treatment results approach maximal levels, consideration must be given to techniques of refining treatment methods without engendering any risk of decreased effectiveness. (This aspect is discussed in a separate section of this chapter.)

The present approaches to patients in various clinical groups (stages) are indicated below:

Group (stage) I (favorable histology): Nephrectomy with no postoperative radiotherapy. Chemotherapy with AMD and VCR for 6 months.

Group (stage) II (favorable histology): Nephrectomy. Postoperative radiotherapy was given in NWTS-2. The actual need for irradiation and the possibility of using less radiation are being explored in NWTS-3 (10). Chemotherapy with AMD, VCR, and ADR is given for 15 months. Intensification of the two-drug regimen is being studied in NWTS-3 to determine if results comparable to the three-drug regimen can be achieved without ADR (10).

Group (stage) III (favorable histology): Nephrectomy. The possibility of lesser postoperative irradiation is being assessed in NWTS-3 (1,000 versus 2,000 rads) (10). Chemotherapy regimens are the same as in group II.

Group (stage) IV and patients with unfavorable histology, all groups: These patients require maximum therapy. Radiotherapy is given postoperatively to tumor bed and metastatic sites. Two schedules of the three-drug (AMD, VCR, and ADR) combination are being studied in NWTS-3 (10).

Histopathology

From analysis of massive amounts of histopathologic data in NWTS-1, certain cytologic features were identified as being associated with unfavorable outcome (1). Although 30 tissue patterns or cell types were recorded for each tumor, two unfavorable histopathologic forms were noted.

One of the unfavorable features was the presence of large, pleomorphic, hyperchromatic nuclei within the tumor cell with abnormal multipolar mitotic figures. The term anaplasia was applied to these tumors (1). The second unfavorable pattern consisted of poorly differentiated stromal cells of the rhabdomyosarcomatoid pattern, clear cell pattern, or hyalinizing pattern (1). The term sarcomatous Wilms' tumor was used to characterize the second pattern.

In terms of disease-free survival and overall survival, there was a significant correlation between the presence or absence of these histopathologic features and outcome of treatment (Table 6). These indicate that 88% of the patients had favorable histology (absence of unfavorable features), and 12% had unfavorable histology. Fifty-two percent of all tumor deaths occurred among those with unfavorable histology, even though only 12% of all patients had unfavorable histology (1). Anaplasia apparently was influenced by age, occurring almost always in the group older than 2 years (24 of 25 cases) (1). The overall tumor death rates among those with favorable histology were 3% under age 2 years (3 of 113) and 9% over age 2 years (137 of 265). The tumor death rate for those with unfavorable histology was 57% (28 of 49).

In addition to the prognostic implications as to treatment fail-

TABLE 6. *Summary of relationship between histopathologic type and survival in 427 patients*

Parameter	No anaplasia		Anaplasia (all ages)	Sarcomas (all ages)
	Under age 2 years	Over age 2 years		
No.	113 (26%)	265 (62%)	25 (6%)	24 (6%)
Relapse-free	108	197	9	5
Tumor death	3	23	14	14
Nontumor death	2	12	0	2

[a] From Beckwith and Palmer (1) and Breslow et al. (5) (NWTS).

ure and mortality, the histopathologic features might predict the biologic behavior of a given tumor. For example, preliminary observations have already suggested that 12 of 13 patients with bone metastases had primary tumors of the distinctive clear cell pattern of the renal sarcoma subtype (1). If metastatic patterns can be predicted, the clinical management of patients could become increasingly more specific.

Age

Age had been recognized in the past as a prognostic factor in survival among patients with Wilms' tumor (58). Although the earlier studies utilized neither prospective staging techniques nor standardized treatment regimens, age seemed to be an important determinant of outcome. Children under 2 years of age had significantly better survival than those over 2 years of age (58) (Table 7).

Results from NWTS have now permitted a more precise assessment of the effect of age on treatment outcome (5,8,58). Those under 2 years of age had a more substantially reduced relapse rate than those over 2 years, even when such other factors as histopathology and extent of disease were taken into consideration (Table 8).

Additional data are obviously required to define more clearly

TABLE 7. *Age versus survival in Wilms' tumor treated before 1970*

	Age under 2 years		Age over 2 years	
Ref.	No. of cases	Survival rate (%)	No. of cases	Survival rate (%)
27	119	41	215	27
22	122	48	213	19
28	75	68	130	48
55	19	63	32	29
55	29	85	56	47

In these patients, no prospective grouping or staging was utilized.

TABLE 8. *Age versus relapse and survival in 429 patients metastasis-free at diagnosis*[a]

Age at diagnosis (years)	No.	Percent relapse	Percent died
0 to 1	135	14.8	10.4
2 to 3	167	34.7	17.4
4+	127	27.6	16.5

[a]From Breslow et al. (5) and D'Angio et al. (8) (NWTS-1).

the interaction between age and treatment on outcome of therapy. For example, in NWTS-1, there was no significant difference in results between the group I cohort that received postoperative radiation therapy and the cohort that did not. When the patients were stratified in terms of age, however, the relapse rate was higher in the older patients (Table 9).

In the second national study, this slight difference caused concern, since all group I patients now received no radiotherapy. In reality, the concern was easily resolved. In the first study, group I patients received only AMD as single agent adjuvant chemotherapy. A more effective double agent chemotherapy regi-

TABLE 9. *Age effect on treatment results in group I patients in NWTS-1*[a]

Age (years)	Radiotherapy[b]	No.	Actuarial proportion at 2 years (+ SE)	
			Disease-free	Surviving
Under 2	Yes	38	0.90 ± 0.06	0.97 ± 0.03
	No	36	0.88 ± 0.06	0.94 ± 0.04
Over 2	Yes	39	0.77 ± 0.07	0.97 ± 0.03
	No	41	0.58 ± 0.08	0.91 ± 0.05

[a]From Breslow et al. (5) and D'Angio et al. (8).
[b]Treatment regimens varied only with respect to postoperative radiotherapy to the tumor bed.

men with AMD and VCR was given in the second study. Preliminary inspection of the data from the second study indicates that among 117 group I patients treated, there have been no relapses recorded, regardless of age (10,43).

It is possible that the development of increasingly more effective treatments and the recognition of prognostically unfavorable cases will eventually minimize the apparent effect of age on outcome.

Other Prognostic Variables

Multivariate statistical analyses of NWTS-1 data have identified several other candidate factors for predicting outcome (5). Significant among them were specimen weight over 250 g and involvement of regional lymph nodes. High correlations were noted between age and specimen weight and between unfavorable histology and lymph node involvement.

Tumor size (indirectly indicated by weight) had been used as a criterion for staging (17), but its significance has been questioned in some studies (22,23).

Lymph nodes were positive in 11% of 350 cases in NWTS-1 (26). When only hilar nodes were involved, disease-free survival was 57%. Disease-free survival rate dropped to 33% when both hilar and aortic nodes were involved (26) (Table 10). Similar

TABLE 10. *Lymph node involvement and outcome*[a]

Pathologic examination	Total	Relapse-free		Alive	
		No.	%	No.	%
Not examined	105	84	80	95	91
Negative	206	149	72	177	86
Hilar nodes positive	30	17	57	22	73
Hilar and aortic nodes positive	9	3	33	3	33
	350				

[a] From Leape et al. (26).

results have been reported from France (28). When regional nodes were obviously or suspiciously involved, the 2- and 5-year survival rates dropped significantly ($p = 0.05$) compared to those with no regional node disease (28). The French data, however, should be evaluated with the knowledge that preoperative irradiation was given in 71% of the patients.

These findings emphasize the deleterious impact of lymph node involvement on relapse-free survival, but data are lacking to assess the therapeutic significance of total periaortic lymphadenectomy (13,26).

GENETIC CONSIDERATIONS

Genetic aspects of Wilms' tumor have been examined recently, with respect to both etiologic implications and genetic counseling for the surviving patient and/or the relatives of the patient.

Knudson and Strong (24,25,49) have proposed a two-step mutation hypothesis for Wilms' tumor, similar to retinoblastoma (24). In the genetic or prezygotic form (30% of unilateral and all bilateral cases) the first mutation is presumed to occur prezygotically. The Wilms' tumor trait in such cases is transmitted as an autosomal dominant gene with 63% penetrance (50,51). The hereditary form tends to occur at an early age, may be multifocal, and is bilateral in 15% (50,51). Tumor does not develop in about 37% of gene carriers. This reduced penetrance implies that unaffected relatives of the hereditary cases may be gene carriers with risk of Wilms' tumor in their offspring (36,50,51).

Based on the above hypothesis, certain statistical projections can be advanced and used for counseling purposes (Table 11). Because of these genetic considerations, the determination of the gene carriers, that is, the population at risk, would be of inestimable benefit. Search should be continued for histopathologic markers, such as multifocal metanephric abnormality found by Bove and McAdams (4) in all patients with bilateral Wilms' tumors and in 14 of 60 patients with unilateral tumors. It has been suggested that the association of Wilms' tumor with certain congeni-

TABLE 11. *Genetic aspects of Wilms' tumor*

Aspect	Percent
Wilms' tumor types	
Nonhereditary (sporadic, postzygotic)	62
Hereditary (dominant gene, prezygotic)	38
Risk of Wilms' tumor in gene carrier	
No tumor	37
Unilateral tumor	48
Bilateral tumor	15
Risk of Wilms' tumor in offspring	
Parent: hereditary case	30
Parent: nonhereditary case	5[a]
Risk of Wilms' tumor in siblings and first cousins	
Hereditary Case	1 to 2

[a] This estimate is lower than the previously published value (50).

tal anomalies, such as aniridia, may be genetically determined (47,50,51). Chromosome markers or linkage association may provide leads to the early diagnosis of gene carriers (35,50–52). For example, chromosomal imbalance in the nature of 11p interstitial deletion has been suggested as one cause for the aniridia–Wilms' tumor association (47,52).

The occurrence of subsequent malignant tumors (of different histologic types) in many surviving Wilms' tumor patients has engendered the suggestion that the hereditary form of Wilms' tumor may be associated with increased risk of such carcinogenesis (36,37,52).

CURRENT ATTITUDES

Bilateral Wilms' Tumor

Concurrent, bilateral renal involvement is seen in approximately 5% of patients with Wilms' tumor (Table 12). Tumor may develop subsequently in the remaining kidney in another 3% of the cases (NWTS-1). The age distribution among 30 children with bilateral Wilms' tumor in NWTS-1 was as follows:

TABLE 12. *Frequency of bilateral Wilms' tumor*

Study	Total no. of patients	No. of bilateral cases	Incidence (%)
NWTS-1 (3)	606	33	5.4
NWTS-2 (43)	374	23	6.1
SIOP (29)	398	13	3.3
	1,378	69	5.0

under 1 year of age, 4; between 1 and 2 years of age, 13; and older than 24 months, 13 (3).

The study protocol for NWTS-1 did not provide therapy guidelines for bilateral cases. Overall survival, however, was surprisingly good. Of 30 patients, 26 (87%) were surviving at 2 years (3). The treatments were individualized and consisted of integrated surgical, radiotherapeutic, and chemotherapeutic approaches.

This experience emphasizes several important aspects of bilateral Wilms' tumor. First, the existence of bilateral involvement was not suspected in one-third of the cases until the contralateral kidney was inspected at the time of operation (3). Bilateral tumor was demonstrated in one-third of the cases by physical findings and in another one-third by IVP. Second, despite varied therapy regimens, survival data are significant. Third, the late effects of therapy, if any, remain to be manifested. Radiation therapy to the only kidney generates apprehension regarding renal function in the future. Finally, all bilateral cases are thought to represent the hereditary type of Wilms' tumor (50,51). The possibility of enhanced susceptibility of the survivor to other cancers must be kept in mind (36,37). The risk of Wilms' tumor in offspring and in relatives of the patient must also be assessed (36,50,51).

Refinement of Therapy

For the first time in cancer therapy, it has become possible in Wilms' tumor to achieve control rates sufficiently high to consider and to actually achieve a reduction in intensity of treatment without a corresponding loss in disease control.

NWTS-1 tested the hypothesis that postoperative radiotherapy would not be necessary if the primary tumor was localized to the kidney and was completely resected (group I patients). A randomized one-half of group I patients in NWTS-1, therefore, did not receive postoperative radiotherapy to the tumor bed (7). These patients had survival results statistically similar to those in group I patients who received postoperative radiotherapy (8,11,16). The results appeared to be clear cut in children under the age of 2 years. In the older age group, fewer infradiaphragmatic relapses and fewer deaths were recorded in the group receiving postoperative radiotherapy. Group I patients in NWTS-1 were given single agent chemotherapy (AMD).

In NWTS-2, postoperative radiotherapy was omitted in all group I patients; the patients received double agent adjuvant chemotherapy (AMD and VCR) (41). In an early analysis, it is reported that no difference in disease-free survival exists among 117 nonirradiated group I patients of all ages followed at least 1 year (43). Thus it is reasonable to assume that children who have Wilms' tumor restricted to the kidney and apparently totally removed surgically (group I) do not require postoperative radiotherapy to the tumor bed.

The question of radiation dosage in other clinical situations (group II and III patients) is undergoing hard evaluation (6, 11,64). Examination of the data from NWTS-1 (11,64) and from other studies (19) suggests that relapse-free survival rates and rad doses may not be correlated. Higher doses did not necessarily provide better control rates (11,19). Lower doses in infants appeared to yield satisfactory results (11). The existence of unfavorable prognostic factors, such as histopathology, appeared to be a significant determinant of prognosis (5). Thus it is possible that current radiotherapy requirements may be refined (and reduced) in the near future.

Early experience with AMD suggested that multiple courses of the drug were therapeutically more desirable than a single course (69,70). Although overall survival statistics showed no significant differences, the multiple course schedule produced fewer relapses (70). This suggested that the survivors who had relapsed from initial single course therapy had to be retrieved with additional treatment (70). The definite possibility that retrieval therapy may not be successful and the risk of potential morbidity associated with additional radiotherapy and chemotherapy clearly indicate the desirability of avoiding the problems if possible.

Based on findings from NWTS-1, NWTS-2 tested in group I patients the hypothesis that two-drug chemotherapy (AMD and VCR) administered for 6 months would be equally as effective as the two drugs given for the traditional 15 months. Preliminary observation of the data suggests that the results of shortened chemotherapy regimen were equally as good as the 15-month regimen (10,43). Because of such experiences, it may not be unreasonable to speculate on the possibility that the recognition of prognostic factors will become increasingly more precise, and that eventually it may be feasible to identify a group of patients who will need surgery alone for treatment.

Modification of Chemotherapy

One of the major results of NWTS-1 has been the demonstration that the combination of AMD and VCR as adjuvant chemotherapy produced significantly better survival results than the use of either drug alone (8). NWTS-1 further showed that under certain circumstances, it has become possible to reduce the intensity of treatment without compromising disease control. However, the same study indicated obvious areas in which improvement of therapy is still necessary; these are patients with prognostically unfavorable clinical presentations (1,5).

The first step has been the evaluation of ADR, a new drug that has demonstrated antitumor activity in patients with metastatic Wilms' tumor (2). There has been the preliminary suggestion that the three-drug combination of ADR with AMD and

VCR is more effective than the two-drug combination of AMD and VCR (10,43). At present, the obvious situations that require the development of more effective therapy regimens include patients with tumors of unfavorable histopathology, patients with group III and IV disease, and patients who fail on primary therapeutic programs.

The concept of preoperative chemotherapy utilizing VCR has been proposed to reduce the size of tumor to facilitate surgery (60). Successful utilization of this approach has already been reported (53). Two or three doses of VCR given 5 days apart (1.5 to 2.0 mg/M^2 per dose) can produce significant reduction in size of Wilms' tumor in most cases (53). Surgery is scheduled about 1 week after the last dose of VCR. Wagget and Koop (67) utilized AMD (single course) or VCR (weekly $\times$ 3 or 4) along with irradiation (1,200 rads in 10 days) preoperatively in children with large tumors. Consistent tumor regression occurred. Although in NWTS-1 preoperative VCR was utilized in metastatic cases (group IV), no meaningful data have been reported (8).

Prognosis After Relapse

Failures of primary treatment in patients with Wilms' tumor are manifested as several types of relapses: recurrence locally (i.e., in the tumor bed), recurrence elsewhere in the abdomen, or metastases to distant sites, such as the lungs, brain, and bone. In addition, there is a special group [about 9% of patients with Wilms' tumor (7)] who have demonstrable metastases at the time of diagnosis. Comparative assessment of most published results of treatment in these patients across therapeutic epochs is not suitable because of the changing therapeutic programs, the continuing development of new effective chemotherapeutic agents, and the identification of prognostic factors. The NWTS-1 (57) has provided for the first time a patient population in which the premetastatic clinical management was controlled. Although the postmetastatic therapy was not rigidly controlled in NWTS-

1, the data provide a more quantitative perspective of the known clinical fact that many patients with metastatic Wilms' tumor will survive (Table 13). The survival rate in groups I and II approximated 45%; the survival rate in group IV patients who had metastases at diagnosis was 56%. The periods of observation on the surviving patients ranged from 1 to 5 years, with the median in excess of 4 years.

Factors that were significantly related to postrelapse survival in group I to III patients were histology, time to relapse, and site of metastasis. Unfavorable histology, early relapse, and metastasis to sites other than lung were bad prognostic features. The patients who were initially group I had significantly better postrelapse survival than those who were initially groups II or III. This difference was caused by metastases being limited to the lungs in most group I patients who relapsed (Table 13).

These results provide more quantitative estimates of the widespread clinical experience that metastatic Wilms' tumor is responsive, in varying degrees, to radiation therapy (42,45), to surgical intervention (62), and to aggressive multimodal therapy (68).

TABLE 13. *Survival after relapse*

Parameter	Initially Group I–III	Initially Group IV
No. of patients	103	84
Surviving	46(45%)	47(56%)
Postmetastatic follow-up time		
Range	1+ to 5+ years	1+ to 5+ years
Median	4+ years	4+ years
Site of metastases		
Lung alone	74	64
Survival	49%	63%
Other sites	29	20
Survival	28%	35%

[a]From Sutow et al. (57).

LATE EFFECTS OF THERAPY

The development of more effective treatment regimens in Wilms' tumor has significantly improved the cure rates and has lengthened the periods of disease control. With the increase in the magnitude of the surviving patient population and in the duration of the survival periods, there have emerged concomitantly problems concerned with therapy-related late effects, including anatomic disturbances, physiologic dysfunctions, oncogenesis, and genetic risks (18,21,30,32–35). The subject matter has broad relevance to pediatric oncology in general; therefore, it is discussed more fully in the chapter on cost of survival.

A perspective of the developing situation is afforded by the analysis of single institutional data on 274 Wilms' tumor patients from the Sidney Farber Cancer Center (Children's Cancer Research Center) for the period from 1945 to 1969 (30,32). For successive quinquennia after 1945, the 3-year survival rates increased steadily: 18, 19, 48, 55, and 67% (32). Among 140 patients alive at 3 years, however, 14 late deaths have occurred (10%). Actuarial analysis projected excess mortality up to 25 years. Mortality after the third year has been attributed chiefly to "sequelae of curative therapy for aggressive lesions" (30,32).

In another review, Everson (14) has reported data from the End Results Group of the National Cancer Institute. Of 225 patients alive 3 years after diagnosis, 12 (6%) died. Diagnosis was made between 1935 and 1969 in these patients. Compiled data, however, tend to obscure the effect of treatment, which has become significantly better with time. Furthermore, without analysis of the actual therapy used at the various institutions providing the data, firm conclusions cannot be drawn. Nonetheless, the existence of late mortality, whatever the magnitude, appears to be established, and the relationship of that mortality to prior therapeutic measures seems ominously direct.

REFERENCES

1. Beckwith, J. B., and Palmer, N. F. (1978): Histopathology and prognosis of Wilms tumor. *Cancer,* 41:1937–1948.

2. Bellani, F. F., Gasparini, M., and Bonadonna, G. (1975): Adriamycin in Wilms's tumor previously treated with chemotherapy. *Eur. J. Cancer,* 11:593–595.
3. Bishop, H. C., Tefft, M., Evans, A. E., and D'Angio, G. J. (1977): Survival in bilateral Wilms' tumor—Review of 30 National Wilms' Tumor Study cases. *J. Pediatr. Surg.,* 12:631–638.
4. Bove, K. E., and McAdams, A. J. (1976): The nephroblastomatosis complex and its relationship to Wilms' tumor: A clinicopathologic treatise. *Perspect. Pediatr. Pathol.,* 3:185–223.
5. Breslow, N. E., Palmer, N. F., Hill, L. R., Buring, J., and D'Angio, G. J. (1978): Wilms' tumor: Prognostic factors for patients without metastases at diagnosis. Results of the National Wilms' Tumor Study. *Cancer,* 41:1577–1589.
6. Cassady, J. R., Tefft, M., Filler, R. M., Jaffe, N., and Hellman, S. (1973): Considerations in the radiation therapy of Wilms' tumor. *Cancer,* 32:598–608.
7. D'Angio, G. J., Beckwith, J. B., Bishop, H. C., Breslow, N., Evans, A. E., Goodwin, W. E., King, L. R., Pickett, L. K., Sinks, L. F., Sutow, W. W., and Wolff, J. A. (1973): The National Wilms' Tumor Study: A progress report. *Seventh National Cancer Conference Proceedings,* pp. 627–636. Lippincott, Philadelphia.
8. D'Angio, G. J., Evans, A. E., Breslow, N., Beckwith, B., Bishop, H., Feigl, P., Goodwin, W., Leape, L. L., Sinks, L. F., Sutow, W., Tefft, M., and Wolff, J. (1976): The treatment of Wilms' tumor. Results of the National Wilms' Tumor Study. *Cancer,* 38:633–646.
9. D'Angio, G. J., Farber, S., and Maddock, C. L. (1959): Potentiation of x-ray effects by actinomycin D. *Radiology,* 73:175–177.
10. D'Angio, G. J., Goodwin, W. E., Ehrlich, R. M., Tefft, M., Beckwith, J. B., and Bishop, H. C. (1978): Wilms Tumor Study. *Dialogues Pediatr. Urol.,* 1(11/12):1–12.
11. D'Angio, G. J., Tefft, M., Breslow, N., and Meyer, J. A. (1978): Radiation therapy of Wilms' tumor: Results according to dose, field, post-operative timing and histology. *Int. J. Radiat. Oncol. Biol. Phys.,* 4:769–780.
12. Editorial (1973): Nephroblastoma: An index reference cancer. *Lancet,* 2:651.
13. Ehrlich, R. M., and Goodwin, W. E. (1973): The surgical treatment of nephroblastoma (Wilms tumor). *Cancer,* 32:1145–1149.
14. Everson, R. B. (1975): Late mortality in Wilms' tumor. *Lancet,* 1:810.
15. Farber, S., D'Angio, G., Evans, A., and Mitus, A. (1960): Clinical studies of actinomycin D with special reference to Wilms' tumor in children. *Ann. NY Acad. Sci.,* 89:421–424.
16. Fraumeni, J. F., Jr., and Glass, A. G. (1968): Wilms' tumor and congenital aniridia. *JAMA,* 206:825–828.
17. Garcia, M., Douglass, C., and Schlosser, J. V. (1963): Classification and prognosis in Wilms's tumor. *Radiology,* 80:574–580.
18. Harris, C. C. (1976): The carcinogenicity of anticancer drugs: A hazard in man. *Cancer,* 37:1014–1023.
19. Hussey, D. H., Castro, J. R., Sullivan, M. P., and Sutow, W. W. (1971):

Radiation therapy in management of Wilms's tumor. *Radiology,* 101:663–668.

20. Innis, M. D. (1973): Nephroblastoma: Index cancer of childhood. *Med. J. Aust.,* 2:322–323.

21. Jaffe, N. (1976): Late side effects of treatment: Skeletal, genetic, central nervous system and oncogenic. *Pediatr. Clin. North Am.,* 23:233–244.

22. Jereb, B., and Eklund, G. (1973): Factors influencing the cure rate in nephroblastoma. *Acta Radiol. (Ther.),* 12:84–106.

23. Jereb, B., and Sandstedt, B. (1973): Structure and size versus prognosis in nephroblastoma. *Cancer,* 31:1473–1481.

24. Knudson, A. G., Jr. (1977): Mutation and cancer in man. *Cancer,* 39:1882–1886.

25. Knudson, A. G., Jr., and Strong, L. C. (1972): Mutation and cancer: A model for Wilms' tumor of the kidney. *J. Natl. Cancer Inst.,* 48:313–324.

26. Leape, L. L., Breslow, N. E., and Bishop, H. C. (1978): The surgical treatment of Wilms' tumor: Results of the National Wilms' Tumor Study. *Ann. Surg.,* 187:351–356.

27. Ledlie, E. M., Mynors, L. S., Draper, G. J., and Gorbach, P. D. (1970): Natural history and treatment of Wilms's tumour: An analysis of 335 cases occurring in England and Wales 1962–6. *Br. Med. J.,* 4:195–200.

28. Lemerle, J., Tournade, M-F., Gerard-Marchant, R., Flamant, R., Sarrazin, D., Flamant, F., Lemerle, M., Jundt, S., Zucker, J-M., and Schweisguth, O. (1976): Wilms' tumor: Natural history and prognostic factors. A retrospective study of 248 cases treated at the Institut Gustave-Roussy, 1952–1967. *Cancer,* 37:2557–2566.

29. Lemerle, J., Voute, P. A., Tournade, M. F., Delemarre, J. F. M., Jereb, B., Ahstrom, L., Flamant, R., and Gerard-Marchant, R. (1976): Preoperative versus postoperative radiotherapy, single versus multiple courses of actinomycin D, in the treatment of Wilms' tumor. Preliminary results of a controlled clinical trial conducted by the International Society of Paediatric Oncology (S.I.O.P.). *Cancer,* 38:647–654.

30. Li, F. P. (1977): Follow-up of survivors of childhood cancer. *Cancer,* 39:1776–1778.

31. Li, F. P. (1978): Host factors in the development of childhood cancers. *Semin. Oncol.,* 5:17–23.

32. Li, F. P., Bishop, Y., and Katsioules, C. (1975): Survival in Wilms' tumour. *Lancet,* 1:41–42.

33. Li, F. P., Cassady, J. R., and Jaffe, N. (1975): Risk of second tumors in survivors of childhood cancer. *Cancer,* 35:1230–1235.

34. Li, F. P., and Stone, R. (1976): Survivors of cancer in childhood. *Ann. Int. Med.,* 84:551–556.

35. Meadows, A. T., D'Angio, G. J., Evans, A. E., Harris, C. C., Miller, R. W., and Mike, V. (1975): Oncogenesis and other late effects of cancer treatment in children. *Radiology,* 114:175–180.

36. Meadows, A. T., Li, F. P., Strong, L. C., Schweisguth, O., and Baum, E. S. (1976): Childhood cancer in siblings. *Pediatr. Res.,* 10:455 (Abstr.).

37. Meadows, A. T., D'Angio, G. J., Miké, V., Banfi, A., Harris, C., Jenkin,

R. D. T., and Schwartz, A. (1977): Patterns of second malignant neoplasms in children. *Cancer,* 40:1903–1911.

38. Medical Research Councils' Working Party on Embryonal Tumours in Childhood (1978): Management of nephroblastoma in childhood. Clinical study of two forms of maintenance chemotherapy. *Arch. Dis. Child.,* 53:112–119.

39. Miller, R. W. (1968): Relation between cancer and congenital defects: An epidemiologic evaluation. *J. Natl. Cancer Inst.,* 40:1079–1085.

40. Miller, R. W., Fraumeni, J. F., Jr., and Manning, M. D. (1964): Association of Wilms's tumor with aniridia, hemihypertrophy, and other congenital malformations. *N. Engl. J. Med.,* 270:922–927.

41. Miller, R. W., Fraumeni, J. F., Jr., and Manning, M. D. (1964): Excessive concurrence of Wilms' tumor with aniridia, hemihypertrophy, and other congenital defects. *J. Pediatr.,* 65:1088–1089.

42. Monson, K. J., Brand, W. N., and Boggs, J. D. (1970): Results of small-field irradiation of apparent solitary metastasis from Wilms's tumor. *Radiology,* 104:157–160.

43. National Wilms' Tumor Study Committee (1978): The National Wilms' Tumor Study. A report from cancer cooperative study groups. *Cancer Clin. Trials,* 1:61–64.

44. Pendergrass, T. W. (1976): Congenital anomalies in children with Wilms' tumor. A new survey. *Cancer,* 37:403–409.

45. Phillips, T. L. (1976): The radiotherapeutic management of pulmonary metastases. *Int. J. Radiat. Oncol. Biol. Phys.,* 1:743–746.

46. Pochedly, C., and Miller, D. (editors) (1976): *Wilms' Tumor.* Wiley, New York.

47. Riccardi, V. M., Sujansky, E., Smith, A. C., and Francke, U. (1978): Chromosomal imbalance in the aniridia—Wilms' tumor association: 11p interstitial deletion. *Pediatrics,* 61:604–610.

48. Silva-Sosa, M., and Gonzalez-Cerva, J. L. (1966): Wilms' tumor in children. *Prog. Clin. Cancer,* 2:323–337.

49. Strong, L. C. (1977): Theories of pathogenesis: Mutation and cancer. In: *Genetics of Human Cancer,* edited by J. J. Mulvihill, R. W. Miller, and J. F. Fraumeni, Jr., pp. 401–415. Raven Press, New York.

50. Strong, L. C. (1977): Genetic considerations in pediatric oncology. In: *Clinical Pediatric Oncology,* second edition, edited by W. W. Sutow, T. J. Vietti, and D. J. Fernbach, pp. 16–32. C. V. Mosby, St. Louis.

51. Strong, L. C. (1976): Genetic and teratogenic aspects of Wilms' tumor. In: *Wilms' Tumor,* edited by C. Pochedly and D. Miller, pp. 63–77. Wiley, New York.

52. Strong, L. C. (1977): Genetic etiology of cancer. *Cancer,* 40:438–444.

53. Sullivan, M. P., Sutow, W. W., Cangir, A., and Taylor, G. (1967): Vincristine sulfate in management of Wilms' tumor. Replacement of preoperative irradiation by chemotherapy. *JAMA,* 202:381–384.

54. Sutow, W. W. (1967): Effective chemotherapy in children with Wilms' tumor. *South. Med. J.,* 60:254–256.

55. Sutow, W. W. (1976): Wilms' tumor. *Methods Cancer Res.,* 13:31–65.
56. Sutow, W. W. (1979): Wilms' tumor—Retrospect and prospect. In: *Proceedings of the American Cancer Society National Conference on the Care of the Child with Cancer,* pp. 62–70. George F. Stickley, Philadelphia.
57. Sutow, W. W., Breslow, N., Palmer, N. F., D'Angio, G. J., and Meyer, J. A. (1979): Prognosis after relapse in children with Wilms' tumor. Results from the First National Wilms' Tumor Study (NWTS-1). *Proc. AACR ASCO,* 20:68 (Abstr.).
58. Sutow, W. W., Gehan, E. A., Heyn, R. M., Kung, F. H., Miller, R. W., Murphy, M. L., and Traggis, D. G. (1970): Comparison of survival curves, 1956 versus 1962, in children with Wilms' tumor and neuroblastoma. *Pediatrics,* 45:800–811.
59. Sutow, W. W., Hussey, D. H., Ayala, A. G., and Sullivan, M. P. (1977): Wilms' tumor. In: *Clinical Pediatric Oncology second edition,* edited by W. W. Sutow, T. J. Vietti, and D. J. Fernbach, pp. 538–568. C. V. Mosby, St. Louis.
60. Sutow, W. W., and Sullivan, M. P. (1965): Vincristine in primary treatment of Wilms' tumor. *Tex. State J. Med.,* 61:794–799.
61. Sutow, W. W., Thurman, W. G., and Windmiller, J. (1963): Vincristine (leucocristine) sulfate in the treatment of children with metastatic Wilms' tumor. *Pediatrics,* 32:880–887.
62. Swenson, O., and Brenner, R. (1967): Aggressive approach to the treatment of Wilms' tumor. *Ann. Surg.,* 166:657–669.
63. Tan, C. T. C., Dargeon, H. W., and Burchenal, J. H. (1959): The effect of actinomycin D on cancer in childhood. *Pediatrics,* 24:544–561.
64. Tefft, M., D'Angio, G. J., and Grant, W., III (1976): Postoperative radiation therapy for residual Wilms' tumor. Review of group III patients in the National Wilms' Tumor Study. *Cancer,* 37:2768–2772.
65. Young, J. L., Jr., Heiss, H. W., Silverberg, E., and Myers, M. H. (1978): Cancer incidence, survival and mortality for children under 15 years of age. *Am. Cancer Soc.,* 16 pp.
66. Young, J. L., Jr., and Miller, R. W. (1975): Incidence of malignant tumors in U.S. children. *J. Pediatr.,* 86:254–258.
67. Wagget, J., and Koop, C. E. (1970): Wilms' tumor: Preoperative radiotherapy and chemotherapy in the management of massive tumors. *Cancer,* 26:338–340.
68. Wara, W. M., Margolis, L. W., Smith, W. B., Kushner, J. H., and deLorimier, A. A. (1974): Treatment of metastatic Wilms' tumor. *Radiology,* 112:695–697.
69. Wolff, J. A., D'Angio, G. J., Hartmann, J. R., Krivit, W., and Newton, W. A., Jr. (1973): Long-term evaluation of single versus multiple dose dactinomycin therapy of Wilms' tumor. *Proc. Am. Assoc. Cancer Res.,* 14:36.
70. Wolff, J. A., Krivit, W., Newton, W. A., Jr., and D'Angio, G. J. (1968): Single versus multiple dose dactinomycin therapy of Wilms's tumor. *N. Engl. J. Med.,* 279:290–294.

7

Childhood Rhabdomyosarcoma

Rhabdomyosarcoma is a major category among malignant solid tumors of childhood. In white children, it represents about one-half of all malignant soft tissue tumors, having an incidence of about 4.5 cases per million population (86). Examination of data from two pediatric cancer centers and from the Manchester (England) Tumour Registry suggests that rhabdomyosarcoma is seen as frequently as neuroblastoma and Wilms' tumor (71,77). In one tabulation, there were 78 children (7.8%) with rhabdomyosarcoma among 1,000 children with malignant neoplastic diseases treated from 1946 to 1966 (71,77). This number represented 13.4% of 579 children with malignant solid tumors in this series.

HISTORIC CONSIDERATIONS

In the first major textbook published on pediatric oncology, which appeared in 1960 (7), the subject of rhabdomyosarcoma was covered in half a page in the chapter, "Various Tumors Limited to Skin and Soft-somatic Tissues." The ineffectiveness of early chemotherapeutic agents was succinctly summarized by the statement that the author had "observed no case in which chemotherapy altered the course of the disease, even temporarily" (8).

A textbook on pediatric pathology published in 1959 (63) included rhabdomyosarcoma in the category of malignant mesenchymal tumors "which have in common a rapid, invariably fatal clinical course with rapid growth of the primary tumor and the ability to metastasize widely at an early stage of the disease" (64). Dealing specifically with rhabdomyosarcoma, the book states: "the particular tumors which have been referred to as rhabdomyosarcoma tend to have a more consistent pattern than the group as a whole, but [we] do not believe that this vague pattern is sufficient basis for differential classification" (64). A second edition of this textbook, published in 1966, repeats these same words (65).

In contrast to these early gloomy appraisals, childhood rhabdomyosarcoma is now considered to be a chemosensitive tumor (25,39–41,66,69,70,72,76), and significantly improved survival statistics have been published (25,31,40,44). In a review of the experience at M. D. Anderson Hospital with 161 patients, 22 with primary involvement of the head and neck (excluding orbit), who received three-drug chemotherapy [vincristine (VCR), actinomycin D (AMD), and cyclophosphamide: VAC] along with irradiation had a disease-free survival rate of 86% at 5 years (44). This survival rate is impressive because almost all these patients represented inoperable situations (biopsy only) with gross residual tumor.

A historic perspective of childhood rhabdomyosarcoma covering the past three decades permits identification of the developments which, in retrospect, can be considered significant milestones in either concepts of the disease or its management:

1. Clinical documentation of the characteristics of rhabdomyosarcoma in children.
2. Histopathologic definition of childhood rhabdomyosarcoma and clarification of the subtypes.
3. Demographic features of rhabdomyosarcoma and clinicopathologic correlation between microscopic characteristics and clinical behavior.
4. Determination of prognostic factors related to outcome of treatment.
5. Radiotherapeutic considerations.
6. Investigations of new drugs, the development of effective adjuvant chemotherapeutic regimens, and integration of chemotherapy into a multimodal therapeutic program.

7. Recognition that response to chemotherapy may be of sufficient degree to allow modification of the intensity of surgery, e.g., conservative excisional surgery instead of exenteration in selected situations.
8. Intergroup Rhabdomyosarcoma Study (IRS), a national effort.

Clinical Characteristics

In 1950, Stobbe and Dargeon (61) provided early clinicopathologic descriptions of childhood rhabdomyosarcoma. In 1961, Pinkel and Pickren (47) emphasized some of the clinical behavior of the tumor. A few years later, Koop and Tewarson (32) reported more clinical information regarding rhabdomyosarcoma of the head and neck in children. Lawrence et al. (36) published data from a clinicopathologic study of embryonal rhabdomyosarcoma which included 42 children. Soule et al. (58) summarized a series which contained 75 children with rhabdomyosarcoma. A systematic characterization of the tumor in children, as well as an assessment of the prognostic factors, were published by Sutow et al. in 1970 (75).

Although rhabdomyosarcoma may arise in soft somatic tissues in many parts of the body, the primary sites of presentation have been conveniently grouped, because of relative frequency of involvement, into several anatomic categories: orbit, extraorbital head and neck, extremities, trunk, genitourinary (GU) organs, perineum, and intraabdominal sites. Among the GU tumors, sarcoma botryoides of the vagina and bladder was singled out early as a recognizable and charactcristic cntity (42,43,54,56).

Histopathology

Enzinger (12) recently summarized the problems slowing the development of a useful and comprehensive classification of soft tissue sarcomas. The impediments to clear understanding of this complex group of tumors have been the comparative rarity of the tumor and "the great variety and wide morphological range of soft tissue sarcomas which reflect the complexity of mesenchymal tissues" (12).

Stobbe and Dargeon (61) first described the embryonal form in 1950. The alveolar rhabdomyosarcoma was initially reported by Riopelle and Thériault (cited in refs. 1 and 2) and was also described later by Enterline and Horn (11) as well as others (13). The botryoid type, including those arising in the bladder and the biliary system, was identified as a descriptive category (27,42,43,56). Pleomorphic rhabdomyosarcoma described by Stout in 1946 (62) appears to be extremely uncommon in the pediatric age group (14).

Widely used currently is the grouping of rhabdomyosarcoma into embryonal, botryoid, alveolar, and pleomorphic types, based on criteria formalized by Horn and Enterline (26).

Chemotherapy

Early intimations that rhabdomyosarcoma may be responsive to chemotherapeutic agents came from clinical trials with AMD in the mid-1950s (57,78). The antitumor activity of both cyclophosphamide (15,21,46,67) and VCR (55,68,73) was demonstrated during the early 1960s in children with metastatic rhabdomyosarcoma.

The three-drug combination of VCR, AMD, and CYT, acronymically designated VAC, and its systematic utilization as adjuvant chemotherapy were established by 1965 at M. D. Anderson Hospital (69). By that time, the requirements for effective adjuvant therapy were formulated as: a chemosensitive tumor, the availability of effective antitumor drugs, and the utilization of additional effective therapeutic modalities (surgery and radiotherapy) (69).

The original VAC regimen was subsequently modified to administer cyclophosphamide in high dose pulses rather than on a daily low dose schedule (15,21). The data on patients treated by these regimens have been reported periodically (9,14,74,84). The most recent analysis indicated that the overall survival rates are holding up (12 of 19 patients), and that the durations of disease-free status are meaningfully long (6.5 to 10 years) even in patients who would now be classified as clinical group III (74).

More recently (in the early 1970s), adriamycin (ADR) used as a single agent (3,50,79,83), or particularly when combined with dimethyltriazenocarboxamide (DTIC) (4,19), demonstrated significant activity against rhabdomyosarcoma.

As a result of these various experiences, a number of intensive and complicated treatment regimens have been evaluated at different cancer centers (17,18,20,31,48,49,85). These developments led to the eventual structuring of the multimodal, multiagent treatment programs being evaluated comparatively as component arms of the IRS (see below).

Prognostic Factors

One of the early efforts to delineate the prognostic factors in childhood rhabdomyosarcoma was published in 1970 (75). Analysis of the survival data on 78 patients indicated that age, histology, primary site, extent of disease, and treatment each had a significant influence on prognosis. The histologic classification in these cases was derived from a careful review of the diagnostic slides (1,2) utilizing criteria outlined by Horn and Enterline (26).

When the patients were grouped by anatomic site of the primary lesion, best prognosis was noted in children with orbital tumors. Primary tumors involving extremities carried a bad prognosis (75). Good survival occurred in children with sarcoma botryoides, whereas those with alveolar rhabdomyosarcoma fared poorly (75). None of the 24 children in this study considered to have extensive or metastatic disease at the outset survived more than 9.5 months from diagnosis. In this analysis, the 36 children who were less than 7 years of age had a significantly better survival experience than the 18 children who were 7 years or older.

INTERGROUP RHABDOMYOSARCOMA STUDY

The first IRS (IRS-I) was conducted between 1972 and 1978, during which time 780 children were studied (40). The study was organized and conducted by a central steering committee, which included representatives from the three major pediatric cooperative groups (Children's Cancer Study Group A, Southwest Cancer Chemotherapy Study Group, and Acute Leukemia Group B) (38–41). The specialties of pediatric oncology, surgery, radiotherapy, pathology, and biostatistics were represented.

The advantages of a national study of rhabdomyosarcoma were considered to be: (a) rapid accumulation of a statistically valid number of patients within a short period of time to eliminate any secular bias regarding a numerically infrequent cancer; (b) assurance of optimum quality control of the incoming data through group discipline and through experience with use of a standard protocol for treatment assignment and patient management; and (c) incorporation of the best and most current thinking and experience from many centers.

Summary of Results: IRS-I

The major results reported to date from the ongoing analysis of IRS-I are summarized in Table 1 (39–41).

1. A schema for the clinical grouping of patients, based on the extent of disease and result of surgical treatment, was formulated as a framework for treatment assignment. The practicality of the approach was demonstrated, and correlation with prognosis was validated.

2. In patients with localized disease completely excised (group I) and treated with three-drug VAC combination, postoperative irradiation of the tumor bed did not offer a therapeutic advantage.

3. In patients with grossly resected tumor but with microscopic residual (group II) given postoperative irradiation, a two-drug combination of AMD and VCR was equally as effective as the three-drug VAC combination. The omission of cyclophosphamide

TABLE 1. *Summary of results: IRS-I[a]*

Clinical group	No. of patients	Chemotherapy regimen	Radio-therapy	Survival at 2 years (%)	
				Disease-free	Overall
I	26	VAC	Given	86	92
	47	VAC	Not given	80	87
II	65	VA	Given	72	80
	65	VAC	Given	72	76
III	116	Pulse-VAC	Given	69	67
	127	Pulse-VAC + ADR	Given	62	63
IV	56	Pulse-VAC	Given	22	32 to 35
	57	Pulse-VAC + ADR	Given	32	

[a] From refs. 39–41.

from any regimen would obviate the risk of acute and/or delayed hemorrhagic cystitis and its sequelae.

4. In patients with gross residual disease (group III) or with metastatic disease (group IV), the three-drug pulse VAC combination was equally as effective as the four-drug combination of pulse VAC plus ADR. There is obvious need for additional investigation to schedule ADR more effectively in combination regimens.

5. The 2-year relapse-free survival rates were projected to be 83% for group I, 72% for group II, 65% for group III, and 28% for group IV.

6. Local recurrences and distant metastases carried an equally poor prognosis.

7. More precise assessments were obtained of the clinical features of the disease and of the behavior of the tumor under treatment.

Clinical Characteristics

In IRS-I, rhabdomyosarcoma occurred distinctly more commonly in males, with a male to female ratio of 1.47 (330/224).

TABLE 2. *Primary sites by clinical group*[a]

| | Group | | | | | |
Site	I	II	III	IV	Total	Percent
Orbit	1	15	36	2	54	10
Other head and neck	9	30	97	21	157	28
Trunk	7	8	15	8	38	7
Extremities	19	31	21	27	98	18
GU	36	28	27	27	118	21
Intrathoracic	1	1	2	10	14	3
GI and hepatic	0	4	8	4	16	3
Perineum-anus	0	5	6	1	12	2
Retroperitoneum	0	8	23	10	41	7
Other	0	0	3	3	6	1
Total	73	130	238	113	554	100

[a]From IRS report updated to November 1978 (40).

Age distribution showed that 67% of the patients were 10 years of age and under, 12% less than 2 years of age, 33% between 2 and 5 years, 22% between 6 and 10 years, 24% between 11 and 15 years, and 9% between 15 and 20 years. The primary sites of the tumors, in descending order of frequency, were head and neck, GU areas, extremity, trunk, retroperitoneum, and miscellaneous sites (see Table 2).

Clinical Grouping

Grouping or staging of the disease in the patient was based on demonstrable extent of the disease and disease residual after initial definitive surgery (38) (see Table 3). Essentially, the same grouping schema is being utilized for IRS-II (28).

Data from IRS-I indicated that the distribution of clinical groups depended, as anticipated, on the anatomic site of the primary lesion (see Table 3). Statistically, there was an inverse correlation between survival and the severity of the grouping designation (see above). Thus best disease-free survival was noted

TABLE 3. *Clinical grouping (staging) of patients: IRS-I[a]*

Group	Disease
I	Localized disease, completely resected: (a) tumor is confined to the muscle or organ of origin, or (b) infiltration outside this structure, but regional nodes are not involved.
II	These are compromised or regional resections of three types, including patients with: (a) grossly resected tumor with microscopic residual, (b) regional disease, completely resected, in which nodes may be involved and/or extension of tumor into an adjacent organ present, or (c) regional disease with involved nodes, grossly resected, but with evidence of microscopic residual.
III	Incomplete resection or biopsy with gross residual disease.
IV	Distant metastatic disease present at onset.

[a] From ref. 38.

in group I cases and the worst in group IV cases. Although all groups did not receive the same treatment, the study design assigned progressively more intense regimens as the extent of disease involvement worsened.

Assignment to a given clinical stage depended considerably on the attitude and aggressiveness of the surgeon. In the review of extremity cases, the operative records of 14 patients placed in group III suggested that 10 of the 14 patients could have been "converted" to group II (and some possibly to group I) "by an extension of the surgical procedure" (24,34). Other data indicate that for some sites, better results are obtained when "total gross resection, rather than incomplete resection, can be accomplished at some point of the treatment schedule" (34).

Histology

The accumulation of an exceedingly large amount of material for histologic review from IRS-I will undoubtedly result in more precise characterization of childhood rhabdomyosarcoma than

TABLE 4. *Histologic types: IRS-I*[a]

Tumor histology	Percent
Embryonal	57
Alveolar	19
Botryoid	6
Pleomorphic	1
Special undifferentiated, type I	4
Special undifferentiated, type II	3
Undifferentiated	10

[a] From ref. 40.

has been possible in the past (16,59). The early results of morphologic evaluation of the primary tumor are tabulated in Table 4. Definitive analysis of the relationship of the histologic type to the clinical features and prognosis and identification of subtypes are currently in progress (16,60).

Meningeal Relapse

One of the early significant findings in IRS-I was the documentation of meningeal extension of tumor in 20 of 57 patients (35%) with primary tumors arising in parameningeal sites (80). Meningeal involvement did not occur with tumors primary at other anatomic sites, although intracranial brain metastases were seen. These parameningeal sites included the nasopharynx, nasal cavity, paranasal sinuses, and middle ear-mastoid area. Of greatest significance was the mortality rate of 90% (18/20) among these patients.

The symptomatology was comparable to that which accompanies central nervous system (CNS) leukemia. A similarity in pathogenesis might be postulated, the process being basically a direct extension of tumor into a pharmacologic sanctuary site with ineffective concentrations of systemically administered drugs. The complication generally occurred early, with median time to development of 5 months and all within 13 months.

The extremely high frequency of its occurrence, the identification of the population at risk, and the almost certain mortality once the complication has developed have directed major attention to this problem in the design of IRS-II (28,51,80).

Criteria for risk of meningeal involvement include: parameningeal primary tumor, abnormality of cranial nerve function, enlargement of neural foramina on radiographs, or evidence of erosion of bone(s) at the base of the skull (51). In these patients, a program of careful cranial radiation, intrathecal medications, and spinal radiation has been recommended (28,51).

Extremity Lesions

In early studies, it was observed that patients with rhabdomyosarcoma arising in extremities had a much poorer prognosis for disease-free survival than patients with primary lesions at other sites (14,31,75). Although some have suggested that combined modality therapy may have improved survival in these patients (52) and that the prognostic significance of anatomic site could be erased by staging (52), the results of IRS-I confirm the bad prognosis noted in the initial observations (24,29). Thus relapses have occurred in 73% of 15 group III patients (23,29). Amputation with immediate and complete control of the primary lesions does not improve the prognosis (29). Other early observations indicated that patients with alveolar rhabdomyosarcoma have poorer outlook for survival (75), and that most extremity lesions are the alveolar type (14,44). In IRS-I, it has been noted that there was a higher incidence of positive regional lymph nodes in extremity cases, especially in lesions of the upper extremity, suggesting dissemination (30).

Data of these types underscore the need to evaluate closely patients with extremity primaries. In particular, those with alveolar rhabdomyosarcoma arising in an extremity are at greatest risk of treatment failure. It has been suggested that while disease dissemination occurs frequently in extremity lesions, the rate of this disease progression is comparatively slow (75).

Radiotherapy

General guidelines for the administration of radiation therapy in childhood rhabdomyosarcoma and the effectiveness of the treatment have been firmly established over the years (5,10,14, 37,82). In IRS-I, the effect on treatment outcome of chemotherapy given before radiation has been evaluated (81). At the time of the analysis, 77 of 95 (81%) had complete or partial response of the tumor, with 15 of 95 patients showing local recurrence or direct extension to adjacent tissues. The results validated earlier experience that multiagent chemotherapy can produce rapid and marked regression of tumor (69,76,84). The study has allayed fears that 6 weeks of chemotherapy preceding radiation may expose the patient to the risk of progression of local disease. Prior chemotherapy in these patients did not compromise the subsequent delivery of radiotherapy.

SURVIVAL AFTER RECURRENCE/METASTASIS

A most ominous clinical factor in rhabdomyosarcoma appears to be the presence of metastases at initial diagnosis or the subsequent development of recurrence or metastasis. The analysis of 83 children with metastatic rhabdomyosarcoma treated between 1953 and 1974 at M. D. Anderson Hospital showed only six survivors living with no evidence of disease activity at 6, 20, 77, 85, 105, and 112 months from time of metastasis (45). The increased propensity of tumors primary in extremities to metastasize (in 18 of 22 patients, 82%) was striking.

Assessments of postmetastatic survival based on retrospectively accumulated data covering long spans of time are unsatisfactory. By necessity, these are evaluations usually of single institution experiences and represent a mosaic of therapeutic philosophies. The large scale IRS is just now publishing preliminary projections of survival statistics following relapse for patients in clinical groups I to IV (40). The survival times following local recurrence or the appearance of metastases seem short, with a median of 27 weeks for those originally groups I and II and 19 to 24 weeks for those initially groups III and IV.

CONSPECTUS

In 1979, childhood rhabdomyosarcoma and its treatment have become better understood, primarily as the result of the IRS. The published results from IRS-I have already impacted meaningfully on the therapeutic concepts. The continuing analyses of IRS-I hold promise of yielding additional significant data, particularly concerning such aspects as sophisticated histopathologic categorization of the tumors and identification of specific prognostic correlations. The major portion of this chapter, therefore, summarizes the results from IRS-I.

The new IRS-II recently activated (28) will delve further into areas where definitive information is lacking. Among the objectives of IRS-II is the effort to improve therapy for certain specific clinical situations. Included among them are: (a) patients who have metastases at diagnosis or in whom metastases develop during treatment, (b) patients with primary lesions involving the extremities, and (c) those with primary lesions in the parameningeal sites.

A long-range objective already being addressed is the integration of multimodal approaches to achieve refinement of therapy. In particular, this effort concerns the modification of intensity of surgery in GU and pelvic tumors. Response to preoperative chemotherapy was frequently of such magnitude that the use of conservative excisional surgery rather than radical exenteration has been reported over the years (6,22,33,53). The initiation of a trial to evaluate this concept (already supported by considerable positive but anecdotal experience from a number of institutions) is a major achievement.

IRS-I has demonstrated a higher than expected incidence of lymphatic metastases from extremity and GU primary sites

(30,35). The clinical significance of this finding will be weighted by its prognostic correlations and eventual translation into surgical attitudes toward lymph node involvement.

REFERENCES

1. Albores-Saavedra, J., Martin, R. G., and Smith, J. L., Jr. (1963): Rhabdomyosarcoma: A study of 35 cases. *Ann. Surg.,* 157:186–197.
2. Albores-Saavedra, J., Butler, J. J., and Martin, R. G. (1965): Rhabdomyosarcoma: Clinicopathologic considerations and report of 85 cases. In: *Tumors of Bone and Soft Tissues,* pp. 349–366. Year Book Medical Publishers, Chicago.
3. Bonadonna, G., Beretta, G., Tancini, G., Brambilia, C., Bajetta, E., DePalo, G. M., LeLena, M., Bellani, F. F., Gasparini, M., Valagussa, P., and Veronesi, U. (1975): Adriamycin studies at the Institute Nazionale Tumori, Milan. *Cancer Chemother. Rep.,* 6(3):231–245.
4. Cangir, A., Morgan, S. K., Land, V. J., Pullen, J., Starling, K. A., and Nitschke, R. (1976): Combination chemotherapy with adriamycin (NSC-123127) and dimethyltriazeno imidazole carboxamide (DTIC) (NSC-45388) in children with metastatic solid tumors. *Med. Pediatr. Oncol.,* 2:183–190.
5. Cassady, J. R., Sagerman, R. H., Tretter, P., and Ellsworth, R. M. (1968): Radiation therapy for rhabdomyosarcoma. *Radiology,* 91:116–120.
6. Clatworthy, H. W., Jr., Braren, V., and Smith, J. P. (1973): Surgery of bladder and prostatic neoplasms in children. *Cancer,* 32:1157–1160.
7. Dargeon, H. W. (1960): *Tumors of Childhood. A Clinical Treatise.* Paul B. Hoeber, New York.
8. Dargeon, H. W. (1960): Rhabdomyosarcoma. In: *Tumors of Childhood. A Clinical Treatise,* pp. 402–404. Paul B. Hoeber, New York.
9. Donaldson, S., Castro, J. R., Wilbur, J. R., and Jesse, R. (1973): Rhabdomyosarcoma of head and neck in children: Combination treatment by surgery, irradiation, and chemotherapy. *Cancer,* 31:26–35.
10. Edland, R. W. (1965): Embryonal rhabdomyosarcoma. *Am. J. Roentgenol. Rad. Ther. Nucl. Med.,* 93:671–685.
11. Enterline, H. T., and Horn, R. C., Jr. (1958): Alveolar rhabdomyosarcoma: A distinctive tumor type. *Am. J. Clin. Pathol.,* 29:356–366.
12. Enzinger, F. M. (1977): Recent developments in the classification of soft tissue sarcomas. In: *Management of Primary Bone and Soft Tissue Sarcomas,* pp. 219–234. Year Book Medical Publishers, Chicago.
13. Enzinger, F. M., and Shiraki, M. (1969): Alveolar rhabdomyosarcoma: An analysis of 110 cases. *Cancer,* 24:18–31.
14. Fernandez, C. H., Sutow, W. W., Merino, O. R., and George, S. L. (1975): Childhood rhabdomyosarcoma: Analysis of coordinated therapy and results. *Am. J. Roentgenol. Rad. Ther. Nucl. Med.,* 123:588–597.
15. Finkelstein, J. Z., Hittle, R. E., and Hammond, G. D. (1969): Evaluations

of a high dose cyclophosphamide regimen in childhood tumors. *Cancer,* 23:1239–1242.

16. Gaiger, A. M., Soule, E. H., and Newton, W. A., Jr. (1980): Pathology of rhabdomyosarcoma. Experience of the Intergroup Rhabdomyosarcoma Study 1972–1978. *Natl. Cancer Inst. Monogr. (in press).*

17. Ghavimi, F., Exelby, P. R., D'Angio, G. J., Cham, W., Lieberman, P. H., Tan, C., Miké, V., and Murphy, M. L. (1975): Multidisciplinary treatment of embryonal rhabdomyosarcoma in children. *Cancer,* 35:677–686.

18. Ghavimi, F., Exelby, P. R., D'Angio, G. J., Whitmore, W. F., Jr., Lieberman, P. H., Lewis, J. L., Jr., Miké, V., and Murphy, M. L. (1973): Combination therapy of urogenital embryonal rhabdomyosarcoma in children. *Cancer,* 32:1178–1185.

19. Gottlieb, J. A., Baker, L. H., Burgess, M. A., Sinkovics, J. G., Moon, T., Bodey, G. P., Rodriguez, V., Rivkin, S. E., Saiki, J., and O'Bryan, R. M. (1975): Sarcoma chemotherapy. In: *Cancer Chemotherapy. Fundamental Concepts and Recent Advances,* pp. 445–454. Year Book Medical Publishers, Chicago.

20. Grosfeld, J. L., Clatworthy, H. W., Jr., and Newton, W. A., Jr. (1969): Combined therapy in childhood rhabdomyosarcoma: An analysis of 42 cases. *J. Pediatr. Surg.,* 4:637–645.

21. Haddy, T. B., Nora, A. H., Sutow, W. W., and Vietti, T. J. (1967): Cyclophosphamide treatment for metastatic soft tissue sarcoma. Intermittent large doses in the treatment of children. *Am. J. Dis. Child.,* 114:301–308.

22. Hays, D. M., and Ortega, J. (1977): Primary chemotherapy in the management of pelvic rhabdomyosarcoma in infancy and early childhood. In: *Adjuvant Therapy of Cancer,* edited by S. S. Salmon and S. E. Jones, pp. 381–387. North-Holland, Amsterdam.

23. Hays, D. M., Lawrence, W., Sutow, W. W., and Tefft, M. (1978): Extremity tumors in the Intergroup Rhabdomyosarcoma Study (IRS): Progress report. *Proc. AACR ASCO,* 19:415 (Abstr.).

24. Hays, D. M., Sutow, W. W., Lawrence, W., Jr., Moon, T. E., and Tefft, M. (1977): Rhabdomyosarcoma: Surgical therapy in extremity lesions in children. *Orthop. Clin. North Am.,* 8:883–902.

25. Heyn, R. M., Holland, R., Newton, W. A., Jr., Tefft, M., Breslow, N., and Hartmann, J. R. (1974): The role of combined chemotherapy in the treatment of rhabdomyosarcoma in children. *Cancer,* 34:2128–2142.

26. Horn, R. C., Jr., and Enterline, H. T. (1958): Rhabdomyosarcoma: A clinicopathological study and classification of 39 cases. *Cancer,* 11:181–199.

27. Horn, R. C., Jr., Yakovac, W. C., Kaye, R., and Koop, C. E. (1955): Rhabdomyosarcoma (sarcoma botryoides) of the common bile duct. *Cancer,* 8:468–477.

28. Intergroup Rhabdomyosarcoma Study Committee: Protocol for IRS-II, activated November 1, 1978, 88 pp.

29. Intergroup Rhabdomyosarcoma Study Committee: Protocol, p. 5.

30. For IRS-II, activated November 1, 1978, p. 52.

31. Jaffe, N., Filler, R. M., Farber, S., Traggis, D. G., Vawter, G. F., Tefft,

M., and Murray, J. E. (1973): Rhabdomyosarcoma in children. Improved outlook with a multidisciplinary approach. *Am. J. Surg.,* 125:482–487.

32. Koop, C. E., and Tewarson, I. P. (1964): Rhabdomyosarcoma of the head and neck in children. *Ann. Surg.,* 160:95–103.

33. Kumar, A. P. M., Wrenn, E. L., Jr., Fleming, I. D., Hustu, H. O., and Pratt, C. B. (1976): Combined therapy to prevent complete pelvic exenteration for rhabdomyosarcoma of the vagina or uterus. *Cancer,* 37:118–122.

34. Lawrence, W., Jr., and Hays, D. M. (1980): Surgical lessons from the Intergroup Rhabdomyosarcoma Study. *Natl. Cancer Inst. Monogr. (in press).*

35. Lawrence, W., Jr., Hays, D. M., and Moon, T. E. (1977): Lymphatic metastasis with childhood rhabdomyosarcoma. *Cancer,* 39:556–559.

36. Lawrence, W., Jr., Jegge, G., and Foote, F. W., Jr. (1964): Embryonal rhabdomyosarcoma. A clinicopathological study. *Cancer,* 17:361–376.

37. Lindberg, R. D. (1969): Rhabdomyosarcoma in children: Treatment and results. In: *Neoplasia in Childhood,* pp. 209–217. Year Book Medical Publishers, Chicago.

38. Maurer, H. M. (1975): The Intergroup Rhabdomyosarcoma Study (NIH): Objectives and clinical staging classification. *J. Pediatr. Surg.,* 10:977–978.

39. Maurer, H. M., Donaldson, M., Gehan, E. A., Hammond, D., Hays, D. M., Lawrence, W., Jr., Lindberg, R., Moon, T., Newton, W., Ragab, A., Raney, B., Ruymann, F., Soule, E. H., Sutow, W. W., and Tefft, M. (1978): Rhabdomyosarcoma in childhood and adolescence. *Curr. Probl. Cancer,* 2:1–36.

40. Maurer, H. M., Donaldson, M., Gehan, E. A., Hammond, D., Hays, D. M., Lawrence, W., Jr., Lindberg, R., Newton, W., Ragab, A., Raney, R. B., Ruymann, F., Soule, E. H., Sutow, W. W., and Tefft, M. (1980): The Intergroup Rhabdomyosarcoma Study—Update November 1978. *Natl. Cancer Inst. Monogr. (in press).*

41. Maurer, H. M., Moon, T., Donaldson, M., Fernandez, C., Gehan, E. A., Hammond, D., Hays, D. M., Lawrence, W., Jr., Newton, W., Ragab, A., Soule, E. H., Sutow, W. W., and Tefft, M. (1977): The Intergroup Rhabdomyosarcoma Study. A preliminary report. *Cancer,* 40:2015–2026.

42. Mostofi, F. K., and Morse, W. H. (1952): Polypoid rhabdomyosarcoma (sarcoma botryoides) of bladder in children. *J. Urol.,* 67:681–687.

43. Ober, W. B., and Edgcomb, J. H. (1954): Sarcoma botryoides in the female urogenital tract. *Cancer,* 7:75–91.

44. Okamura, J., and Sutow, W. W. (1977): Childhood rhabdomyosarcoma. Clinical aspects of 161 cases. *Shonika Shinryo,* 40:561–568.

45. Okamura, J., Sutow, W. W., and Moon, T. E. (1977): Prognosis in children with metastatic rhabdomyosarcoma. *Med. Pediatr. Oncol.,* 3:243–251.

46. Pinkel, D. (1962): Cyclophosphamide in children with cancer. *Cancer,* 15:42–49.

47. Pinkel, D., and Pickren, J. (1961): Rhabdomyosarcoma in children. *JAMA,* 175:293–298.

48. Pratt, C. B., Hustu, H. O., Fleming, I. D., and Pinkel, D. (1972): Coordi-

nated treatment of childhood rhabdomyosarcoma with surgery, radiotherapy, and combination chemotherapy. *Cancer Res.,* 32:606–610.

49. Pratt, C. B., James, D. H., Jr., Holton, C. P., and Pinkel, D. (1968): Combination therapy including vincristine for malignant solid tumors in children. *Cancer Chemother. Rep.,* 52:489–495.

50. Ragab, A. H., Sutow, W. W., Komp, D. M., Starling, K. A., Lyon, G. M., Jr., and George, S. (1975): Adriamycin in the treatment of childhood solid tumors. *Cancer,* 36:1572–1576.

51. Raney, R. B., Jr., Donaldson, M. H., Sutow, W. W., Lindberg, R. D., Maurer, H. M., and Tefft, M. (1980): Special considerations related to primary site in rhabdomyosarcoma: Experience of the Intergroup Rhabdomyosarcoma Study. *Natl. Cancer Inst. Monogr. (in press).*

52. Ransom, J. L., Pratt, C. B., and Shanks, E. (1977): Childhood rhabdomyosarcoma of the extremity: Results of combined modality therapy. *Cancer,* 40:2810–2816.

53. Rivard, G., Ortega, J., Hittle, R., Nitschke, R., and Karon, M. (1975): Intensive chemotherapy as primary treatment for rhabdomyosarcoma of the pelvis. *Cancer,* 36:1593–1597.

54. Rutledge, F., and Sullivan, M. P. (1967): Sarcoma botryoides. *Ann. NY Acad. Sci.,* 142:694–708.

55. Selawry, O. S., Holland, J. F., and Wolman, I. J. (1968): Effect of vincristine on malignant solid tumors in children. *Cancer Chemother. Rep.,* 52:497–500.

56. Shackman, R. (1954): Sarcoma botryoides of the genital tract in female children. *Br. J. Surg.,* 38:26–30.

57. Shaw, R. K., Moore, E. W., Mueller, P. S., Frei, E., III, and Watkin, D. M. (1960): The effect of actinomycin D on childhood neoplasms. *Am. J. Dis. Child.,* 99:628–635.

58. Soule, E. H., Mahour, G. H., Mills, S. D., and Lynn, H. B. (1968): Soft-tissue sarcomas of infants and children: A clinicopathologic study of 135 cases. *Mayo Clin. Proc.,* 43:313–326.

59. Soule, E. H., and Newton, W. A. (1976): Intergroup Rhabdomyosarcoma Study (IRS). Identification of a histologic subgroup: questionable Ewing's sarcoma of soft tissue. *Proc. AACR ASCO,* 7:301 (Abstr.).

60. Soule, E. H., Newton, W., Jr., Moon, T. E., and Tefft, M. (1978): Extraskeletal Ewing's sarcoma: A preliminary review of 26 cases encountered in the Intergroup Rhabdomyosarcoma Study. *Cancer,* 42:259–264

61. Stobbe, G. D., and Dargeon, H. W. (1950): Embryonal rhabdomyosarcoma of the head and neck in children and adolescents. *Cancer,* 3:826–836.

62. Stout, A. P. (1946): Rhabdomyosarcoma of skeletal muscle. *Ann. Surg.,* 123:447–472.

63. Stowens, D. (1959): *Pediatric Pathology.* Williams & Wilkins, Baltimore.

64. Stowens, D. (1959): In: *Pediatric Pathology,* p. 140. Williams & Wilkins, Baltimore.

65. Stowens, D. (1966): *Pediatric Pathology,* second edition. Williams & Wilkins, Baltimore.

66. Sutow, W. W. (1965): Chemotherapy in childhood cancer (except leukemia): An appraisal. *Cancer,* 18:1585–1589.
67. Sutow, W. W. (1967): Cyclophosphamide in Wilms' tumor and rhabdomyosarcoma. *Cancer Chemother. Rep.,* 51:407–409.
68. Sutow, W. W. (1968): Vincristine therapy for malignant solid tumors in children. *Cancer Chemother. Rep.,* 52:485–487.
69. Sutow, W. W. (1969): Chemotherapeutic management of childhood rhabdomyosarcoma. In: *Neoplasia in Childhood,* pp. 201–208. Year Book Medical Publishers, Chicago.
70. Sutow, W. W. (1970): Drug therapy and curability of childhood cancer. *Postgrad. Med.,* 48:173–177.
71. Sutow, W. W. (1973): General aspects of childhood cancer. In: *Clinical Pediatric Oncology,* edited by W. W. Sutow, T. J. Vietti, and D. J. Fernbach, pp. 1–6. C. V. Mosby, St. Louis.
72. Sutow, W. W. (1977): Perspectives in the management of osteosarcoma and rhabdomyosarcoma in children. In: *Management of Primary Bone and Soft Tissue Tumors,* pp. 25–34. Year Book Medical Publishers, Chicago.
73. Sutow, W. W., Berry, D. H., Haddy, T. B., Sullivan, M. P., Watkins, W. L., and Windmiller, J. (1966): Vincristine sulfate therapy in children with metastatic soft tissue sarcoma. *Pediatrics,* 38:465–472.
74. Sutow, W. W., Fujimoto, T., Wilbur, J. R., and Okamura, J. (1977): Long-term evaluation of VAC chemotherapy in childhood rhabdomyosarcoma. *Proc. AACR ASCO,* 18:291 (Abstr.).
75. Sutow, W. W., Sullivan, M. P., Ried, H. L., Taylor, H. G., and Griffith, K. M. (1970): Prognosis in childhood rhabdomyosarcoma. *Cancer,* 25:1384–1390.
76. Sutow, W. W., and Sullivan, M. P. (1970): Successful chemotherapy for childhood rhabdomyosarcoma. *Tex. Med.,* 66:1–4.
77. Sutow, W. W., and Sullivan, M. P. (1976): Childhood cancer: The improving prognosis. *Postgrad. Med.,* 59:131–137.
78. Tan, C. T. C., Dargeon, H. W., and Burchenal, J. H. (1959): The effect of actinomycin D on cancer in childhood. *Pediatrics,* 24:544–561.
79. Tan, C., Rosen, G., Ghavimi, F., Haghbin, M., Helson, L., Wollner, N., and Murphy, M. L. (1975): Adriamycin in pediatric malignancies. *Cancer Chemother. Rep.,* 6(3):259–266.
80. Tefft, M., Fernandez, C., Donaldson, M., Newton, W., and Moon, T. E. (1978): Incidence of meningeal involvement by rhabdomyosarcoma of the head and neck in children: A report of the Intergroup Rhabdomyosarcoma Study (IRS). *Cancer,* 42:253–258.
81. Tefft, M., Fernandez, C. H., and Moon, T. E. (1977): Rhabdomyosarcoma: Response with chemotherapy prior to radiation in patients with gross residual disease. *Cancer,* 39:665–670.
82. Tefft, M., and Jaffe, N. (1973): Sarcoma of the bladder and prostate in children—Rationale for role of radiation therapy based on a review of the literature and a report of fourteen additional patients. *Cancer,* 32:1161–1177.

83. Wang, J. J., Holland, J. F., and Sinks, L. F. (1975): Phase II study of adriamycin in childhood solid tumors. *Cancer Chemother. Rep.,* 6(3):267–270.
84. Wilbur, J. R., Sutow, W. W., and Sullivan, M. P. (1974): The changing treatment of rhabdomyosarcoma in children, particularly in treatment of inoperable rhabdomyosarcoma of the nasopharynx and oropharynx. In: *Neoplasia of Head and Neck,* pp. 281–288. Year Book Medical Publishers, Chicago.
85. Wilbur, J. R., Sutow, W. W., Sullivan, M. P., and Gottlieb, J. A. (1975): Chemotherapy of sarcomas. *Cancer,* 36:765–769.
86. Young, J. L., Jr., and Miller, R. W. (1975): Incidence of malignant tumors in U.S. children. *J. Pediatr.,* 86:254–258.

8

Ewing's Sarcoma

Ewing's tumor still confronts the oncologist with a sequence of difficult problems. The insidious onset of symptoms frequently delays the institution of proper diagnostic procedures. The pathologist may have difficulty in establishing a definitive diagnosis even when a good biopsy specimen has been obtained. The treatment is multimodal, complex, intensive, and prolonged. Delayed relapses or late metastases preclude early prognostic assessment. Only recently has there been some suggestion that therapy may be improving the survival rates (8,16,22,24,32,38). Finally, the risk of late deleterious effects of therapy is prominent among the surviving patients.

Until major breakthroughs occur in such aspects as the understanding of the tumor, the development of more effective therapy, elimination of late failures, and prevention of delayed effects of therapy, reviews such as this add little to the abundance of published literature on the subject of Ewing's sarcoma.

At this writing, it seems that the concerted efforts of the Intergroup Ewing's Sarcoma Study (IESS) (31,32) should eventually provide the best data for evaluation of the disease. The IESS programs, however, were initiated in 1973 (31) and must mature much longer to yield sufficient 5- and 10-year survival data for firm clinical assessment of therapeutic capabilities.

Therefore, only summary tabulations of data from selected recent reports are presented in this chapter to indicate the clinical characteristics of Ewing's sarcoma and the nature of some problems being investigated at this time (1979).

149

CLINICAL CHARACTERISTICS

Incidence

Data from the Third National Cancer Survey (47) and from the Surveillance, Epidemiology and End Results (SEER) program (48) indicate that Ewing's sarcoma constituted from 1.4% (47) to 1.8% (48) of all malignant neoplasms that occurred in white children under 15 years of age. The incidence of Ewing's sarcoma in white children was 1.7 (48) to 2.1 (47) per million population. When only malignant solid tumors were considered, Ewing's sarcoma accounted for 2.4% (47) to 3.2% (48) of all solid tumors in white children.

A better clinical perspective may be obtained if the incidence of Ewing's sarcoma is compared to the rate of occurrence of more frequently seen solid tumors. Thus viewed, for each case of Ewing's sarcoma in a white child under age 15, the numbers of cases of other selected solid tumors were as follows: central nervous system (brain) tumor, 14.2; neuroblastoma, 5.6; Wilms' tumor, 4.5; soft tissue sarcoma, 5.0 (rhabdomyosarcoma, 2.7); and, osteosarcoma, 2.0 (47).

Age

The calculations of age distribution, while seemingly straight-forward, may require careful examination of the data for hidden biases. For example, the protocols for IESS do not specify any age limit for patient eligibility in the studies (20,21); however, the conduct of the program has a strong pediatric orientation. The genesis of the study was a pediatric activity, and the major participants represented pediatric hospitals and pediatric departments. The accumulated data accordingly should give precise information regarding the tumor within the pediatric population but may yield erroneous answers when extrapolated to the general population. In the IESS report, 70% of 257 patients (32) were 15 years of age or less. The more representative experience at

TABLE 1. *Relative incidence by age in pediatric patients (15 years of age and younger) in IESS[a]*

Age (years)	No.	Percent
Under 6	24	13.1
6 to 10	57	31.1
11 to 15	102	55.7
	183[b]	

[a] From ref. 32.

[b] This number represents 69.8% of 262 patients entered on study.

Mayo Clinic indicated that less than 50%[1] of 299 patients were 15 years or younger (11).

Although Dahlin (11) and Huvos (19) both provide informative histograms of age distribution, accurate readings for specific age groups are difficult. Dahlin's graph (11) indicates that 2 to 3% of the patients were younger than 10 years, and that about 45% were between 10 and 20 years. The histogram by Huvos (19) suggests that more than 30% were in the "first decade" of life and somewhat more than 50% were in the "second decade."

Within the "pediatric" age group (15 years or younger), the IESS data (32) provide a good breakdown of age distribution, as shown in Table 1.

In Dahlin's series (11), the youngest patient was 18 months old. Coley et al. (9) have reported the occurrence of this tumor in an infant 5 months of age.

Sex

Practically all series have shown a male preponderance in the occurrence of Ewing's sarcoma. In 1967, Falk and Alpert (15) reviewed the earlier literature and reported an average M:F ratio

---

[1] Estimated roughly from histogram (11).

TABLE 2. *Sex ratio in Ewing's sarcoma*

Source	No. of patients M	F	M:F ratio
IESS (32)	159	103	1.54
Dahlin (11)	174	125	1.39
Huvos (19)	101	66	1.53
	434	294	1.48

of 1.5 in their collected series of 944 published cases. The sex ratios found in more recent series are indicated in Table 2. The overall M:F ratio was 1.48 in 728 cases.

Race

From a study of death certificates and hospital charts of 482 children dying with the diagnosis of Ewing's sarcoma from 1960 to 1966, Glass and Fraumeni (18) emphasized the virtual absence of nonwhites in the series. Data from the Third National Cancer Survey (47) and from the SEER program (48) substantiate the infrequency of occurrence of Ewing's sarcoma in blacks. Although the rare development of this tumor in black children is occasionally reported (17,23,28,40), the infrequency of this occurrence would almost exclude its consideration in the differential diagnosis of a bone neoplasm in the black population (46).

Primary Site

The site of the primary tumor has been correlated with prognosis in the patient with Ewing's sarcoma. Pritchard et al. (36) reported that the 5-year survival rate was significantly better in those with primary tumor within an extremity. Pomeroy and Johnson (35) noted that the best survival occurred when the tumor involved "peripheral" long bones (below knee and elbow) and the mandible. The next best survival rate was seen in those

TABLE 3. *Anatomic distribution of primary sites in Ewing's sarcoma*

Primary sites	IESS (32) (N = 262)	Dahlin (11) (N = 299)	Huvos (19) (N = 167)	Combined (N = 728)	
				No.	%
Extremities	158	170	106	434	60
Pelvis	50	53	30	133	18
Ribs	17	23	16	56	8
Other	37	53	15	105	14

with primary lesion of the "central" long bones (femur and humerus). The worst prognosis for survival was noted in patients with "trunk" lesions (pelvis, ribs, sternum, and scapula). Data from IESS have indicated that unfavorable prognostic factors included primary lesion in the pelvis or in "proximal sites" (5).

Data showing major categories of primary sites for Ewing's sarcoma have been compiled in Table 3 from several reports of large series. It should be noted that the reports contained varying proportions of different age groups. No effort was made to determine whether or not the frequency distribution of primary sites differed between children and adults. When the statistics from the disparate sources were combined, the tumor arose in an extremity bone in 60% of the cases. The next most common site of involvement was the pelvis (19%).

The data from Dahlin (11) and Huvos (19) allow examination of the relative frequencies with which specific bones were involved (Table 3). Among bones of the extremities, the femur was most frequently involved (24%), followed by humerus (10%), tibia (9%), and fibula (7%). This distribution was comparable to that reported earlier by Falk and Alpert (14).

TREATMENT AND RESULTS

Current treatment programs for Ewing's sarcoma are multimodal (22,34,37), incorporating high-dose radiation therapy, intensive multidrug chemotherapy, and expanded surgical interventions. There is a growing consensus among investigators with wide clinical experiences that the prognosis in patients with Ewing's sarcoma has improved as the result of these therapeutic strategies (22,37). Yet the data do not support this clinical impression as firmly as might be desired. The major deficiencies of the supporting data are one or more of the following:

(1) The numbers of patients treated are inadequate. Conclusions have been derived from less than 10 cases in some reports.
(2) Except for IESS, concurrent randomized trials have not been conducted. Comparisons are made with historic data.
(3) Too long a time span has been required to accumulate enough cases for analysis. Major changes in therapeutic attitudes may have occurred.
(4) The follow-up period has been too short. Some reports include significant numbers of cases with follow-ups of even less than 1 year. (Even the report from IESS does not have sufficient numbers of patients who have been observed for a minimum of 5 years.)

In this section, therefore, it is justifiable only to outline the types of treatments that are being used and to summarize some of the results as reported. For the most part, only publications that have appeared in 1975 or later have been reviewed.

Surgery

Until recently, the programs for the primary management of patients with Ewing's sarcoma generally considered surgery to be of secondary importance, except for purposes of biopsy (4). An occasional amputation was carried out when it appeared probable that postirradiation changes would bring about intolerable functional disability, such as primary involvement of the calcaneus.

Pritchard et al. (36) studied the clinical aspects of 37 long-term survivors among 234 patients with Ewing's sarcoma treated at Mayo Clinic between 1912 and 1968. Location of the primary tumor within an extremity and inclusion of surgery as part of the initial treatment were identified as significant determinants of survival. Surgery generally consisted of amputation, but wide excision was used occasionally. Of 70 patients whose treatment programs included surgery, 34% were surviving at 5 years. In 124 patients treated with no surgery, the 5-year survival rate was 11%. When extremity primaries only were considered, the 5-year survival rates were 45% of 47 patients with surgery and 13% of 61 patients without surgery.

In the protocols for the continuing IESS programs (20,21), it is stated that the preliminary analysis of the data from the initial study seemed to indicate that the time to relapse experience was superior in patients undergoing surgical resection. When both local recurrence and metastases were considered, the failure rate was 7% when partial or complete resection was performed and 29% in those who had no surgical procedure. The study also showed that of patients surviving more than 1 year, "no patient with an incomplete or partial resection died and 42/45 patients are still alive" (20,21).

Based on such available information, the IESS has recommended resection for lesions in expendable bones (21). Amputation is recommended for certain lower extremity primary tumors (unmanageable huge destructive lesion; pathologic fracture; or distal femoral or other distal lesions in children under 6 years where postradiation growth disturbances can be anticipated). With respect to primary involvement of the pelvis and sacrum, complete surgical resection with adequate margins is recommended where possible. Even where total resection is not possible, it is recommended that tumor bulk be reduced as much as possible to decrease "the amount of anoxic tissue present prior to radiation therapy" (20,21).

While statistical data argue in favor of surgical considerations, surgery (such as amputation) affects only the local tumor. If local control can be attained in 95 to 98% of the patients without surgery, the entire question of surgery in Ewing's sarcoma needs careful evaluation. The reduction of tumor mass for irradiation purposes would benefit the patient only if this would permit the use of lesser radiation doses over smaller volume (thereby reducing the risk of radiation-associated late effects). Is it possible that the presence of the primary tumor mass during the weeks of radiation treatment can remain a source of metastases even with concomitant chemotherapy? Does the response to radiation treatment itself cause disruption of tumor sufficient to disseminate microemboli? These are conceptual possibilities, and if they exist, surgery would obviate the danger. Pritchard et al. (36) report that there were no 5-year survivors in 16 patients with Ewing's sarcoma of the ribs. It would seem probable that rib lesions surely would be subjected to attempts at complete surgical excision. The poor outcome suggests the need to delve further into factors that determine the spread of tumor.

Radiotherapy

The basic guidelines developed over a period of years at M. D. Anderson Hospital (8,16,41) will serve as an example of an effective radiation therapy program for Ewing's sarcoma:

(1) Radiation therapy begins as early as possible and is given concurrently with chemotherapy.
(2) The entirety of the involved bone is treated with parallel-opposed fields to administer 4,400 rads tumor dose in 4.5 weeks. Shaped fields are used.
(3) The fields are then reduced to include clinically and radiographically evident tumor for an additional 1,600 rads to give a final dose of 6,000 rads in 6 weeks.

The radiotherapy requirements in the IESS regimens (20,21) prescribe 4,500 rads to the whole bone, 5,000 rads to reduced field (5 cm margin in all directions), and 5,500 rads to the primary tumor (1 cm margin in all directions). The daily dose is 200 rad midplane, five fractions per week. A lesion surgically resected but with microscopic residual is given 5,000 rads total. If the tumor is surgically resected with no microscopic residual, no radiation therapy is administered.

The formulation of radiotherapy guidelines and the development of chemotherapy programs overlapped chronologically. The reports of these studies (summarized in Table 4) included data from varying therapeutic periods. Tefft et al. (43) and Chabora et al. (7) reviewed the published experiences with radiation therapy before the use of intensive systemic chemotherapy. In the seven reports examined, the local control rates (in a total patient population of 150) ranged from 44 to 77%, with an average of 60%.

The most recent update of the results attained at M. D. Anderson Hospital (8) indicates a local control rate of 97% in 36 patients treated with irradiation and chemotherapy between 1969 and 1975. The minimum follow-up time in these patients was 26 months, suggesting that a few were still at risk for local recurrence. In comparison, the preliminary results reported from IESS (33) indicated a local control rate of 87% (of 187 patients) with a median follow-up time of 24 to 30 months. It was noted that 22 of 25 local failures (88%) appeared within 24 months. These analyses of the M. D. Anderson Hospital and IESS data did not separate out categories by primary site but included them all. In the IESS report (33), the median follow-up times for the patients varied from 23 to 37 months for different treatment arms. It remains possible, therefore, to see additional local recurrences as more time elapses.

It should be kept in mind, however, that the precise assessment of the success rate in achieving local control is complicated by the possibility that many patients may die of metastatic disease before local failures become manifest. Also, patients dying of metastatic disease may not have pathologic examination of the primary site. In the early analysis of 187 patients in the IESS

TABLE 4. Summary of reported radiotherapy programs for Ewing's sarcoma

Ref.	Period of study	No. of cases	Radiation dose	Chemotherapy[a]	Results	
					Local failure rate	Survival
8	1948–1964	25	4,000–6,000 rads in 4 to 6 weeks	None	11/25	2/25 (over 18 years)
	1964–1969	15	6,000–7,000 rads in 6 to 7.5 weeks	None	5/15	0/15
	1969–1972	21	6,500–7,000 rads in 6.5 to 7 weeks	VCR, CYT	0/21	10/21 (all over 5 years)
	1973–1976	15	6,000 rads in 6 weeks	VCR, CYT, AMD, ADR	1/15	9/15 (26 to 60 months; median, 37 months)
38	1973–1975	20	6,000–7,000 rads	VCR, CYT, AMD, ADR, (T-2)	5/23[b]	15/20 NED (31 to 82 months; median, 46 months)
	1975–Present	13	6,000–7,000 rads	T-6 induction, AMD, MTX, CYT, VCR, Bleo, ADR, BCNU, T-2 maintenance	[c]	11/13 NED (12 to 26 months; median, 20 months)
22	1950–1975	40	Not stated	Various single agent regimens at most	Not stated	27%
	1971–1975	9	5,500–6,000 rads	VCR, AMD, CYT	2/14[d]	7/9 (4 months to 4.5 years; median 3 years)
3	1960–1970	40	4,500–5,000 rads in 5 to 7 weeks	None	5/40	2/40 (4 years)[d]
	1972–1976	37	4,500–5,000 rads in 5 to 7 weeks	VCR, CYT, ADR	9/37	24/37 (12 to 62 months; average, 29 to 34 months)

[a] MTX, methotrexate; Bleo, bleomycin.
[b] Includes three patients with metastases at diagnosis.
[c] No local failure mentioned.
[d] Includes patient with metastases at diagnosis.

(33), there were 10 local recurrences as the first site of relapse and 15 additional cases in which local recurrence was found concurrently with distant metastases.

Rosen et al. (38) have warned recently against the indiscriminate conclusion that the combination of intensive chemotherapy with irradiation has improved the local control rate in Ewing's sarcoma. They report a local recurrence rate of 22% (5/23) in their series, all failures being noted 18 to 27 months after start of therapy. They suggest that the development of local recurrence had been merely delayed and that eventually the local failure rate may approach that noted during prechemotherapy era. While that possibility exists, it could be pointed out also that the minimum follow-up time in all cases reported by Chan et al. (8) exceeded 26 months.

Chemotherapy

The optimum chemotherapy regimen for Ewing's sarcoma is yet to be developed (42). The ideal regimen will combine the following characteristics: (a) contribute in a major way to disease free survival in 95% or more of the patients with nonmetastatic disease, (b) have maximum patient tolerance and minimum toxicity, (c) allow refinement of other therapeutic modalities, particularly with respect to radiotherapy, and (d) improve overall survival in patients who have metastases at diagnosis and in patients who manifest metastasis during or after treatment.

The current clinical trials are being conducted to identify the drugs with antitumor activity against Ewing's sarcoma, to determine the combinations, doses, sequence, and scheduling of multidrugs, and to optimize the strategy of chemotherapy in conjunction with irradiation and surgery.

Table 5 briefly outlines some of the chemotherapy programs presently being investigated. The reader should study the original publications for detailed and specific information concerning the various regimens. All are in the developmental phase with less than optimal survival results.

TABLE 5. *Current chemotherapy programs for Ewing's sarcoma*

Investigators	Chemotherapy[a]	No. of patients	Results
IESS (32)	VAC + ADR (Regimen 1)	117	74% actuarial RFS[b] at 2 years
IESS (32)	VAC (Regimen 2)	68	35% actuarial RFS at 2 years
IESS (32)	VAC + pulmonary irradiation (Regimen 3)	79	58% actuarial RFS at 2 years
Rosen et al. (38)	VAC + ADR (T-2)	20	75% RFS at 5 years
Rosen et al. (38)	T-6 induction VCR MTX AMD Bleo CYT BCNU ADR T-2 maintenance	13	11/13 disease free at 12 to 26 months
IESS (20,21)	High-dose intermittent schedule (VAC + ADR) (exclude pelvic and sacral primaries)	—	Study in progress
IESS (20,21)	Moderate dose continuous schedule (VAC + ADR) (exclude pelvic and sacral primaries)	—	Study in progress
IESS (20,21)	High-dose intermittent schedule (preoperative, preradiotherapy, postoperative); for pelvic and sacral primaries	—	Study in progress

[a] VAC, three-drug combination of VCR, AMD, and CYT used in varying schedules and doses.
[b] Relapse-free survival.

MISCELLANEOUS COMMENTS

Late Relapses

The best quantitative estimate of the risk of late relapses (after 5 years) comes from the large experience at Mayo Clinic reported by Pritchard et al. (36). In this series of 229 patients, 37 were surviving at 5 years. Of the 37, eight died subsequently of tumor (two between 5 and 6 years, two at 6 years, and one each at 9, 10, 13, and 17 years). The failure rate, therefore, was 21% of those surviving disease-free at 5 years. It would seem justifiable to accept this Mayo Clinic experience as the best available baseline (albeit historic) data.

A number of years ago, Falk and Alpert (15) had examined data on 320 patients compiled from the literature, among whom there were 91 survivors at 5 years. In 18 of these 91 (14%), metastases developed. It is also important to note that 23% (165/720) of the source cases were treated at Mayo Clinic and presumably would be included in the later report by Pritchard et al. (36). The challenge to new therapy then would include the elimination of the late relapses.

Survival After Metastases

Discussions about metastatic Ewing's sarcoma separate into two distinct categories: first, those regarding the patients who are metastatic at diagnosis, and second, discussions about those who develop metastases during or after primary therapy.

Fifteen percent (36) to 35% (34) of patients with Ewing's sarcoma already have metastases at the time of diagnosis. Even with the intensive, multimodal therapy now being used, 25% (38) to 42% (32) or more of those who are apparently disease-free will develop metastases subsequently. The therapeutic implications are significantly different for these two categories of patients.

The frequency of patients with metastases at diagnosis can be expected to vary with the numbers of cases included in the series, with the types of patients usually seen at the particular institution, and with the nature and extent of the diagnostic search for metastases. The presence of metastases suggests widespread, advanced, or rapidly progressive disease. On the other hand, from the therapeutic standpoint, these are patients who have had no previous treatment. All options are available, and all modalities can be used at full intensity.

Data from IESS (45) provide some indication regarding the potential effectiveness of current therapy of previously untreated Ewing's sarcoma. A total of 44 patients with metastases at diagnosis were treated utilizing a common protocol. The patients received radiation therapy to the primary lesion (basic dose of 3,500 rads) as well as to the demonstrable metastases. Chemotherapy included vincristine (VCR), cyclophosphamide (CYT), actinomycin D (AMD), and adriamycin (ADR).

The median duration of time on study for these patients was 75 weeks when analysis was done. Complete regression of tumor occurred in 31 patients (70%); 17 patients (39%) were disease-free, with a median time on study of 21 months (range, 15 to 34 months). The intensity of the therapy regimen is suggested by the occurrence of four deaths (9%) due to toxicity (two from infection and two from ADR cardiomyopathy). These patients were treated from 1975 to 1977. The inadequate durations of follow-up in these patients preclude any prognostic conclusions as to ultimate survival.

Johnson and Pomeroy (24) reported an actuarial survival of 35% at 3 years in 23 patients metastatic at diagnosis. In a subsequent publication (34), the actuarial survival at 4 years for the 23 patients has been depicted as zero. Rosen et al. (38) achieved complete regression of all tumors in eight of eight patients with metastatic Ewing's sarcoma, but only one patient remained disease-free (64 months). The rest relapsed 4 to 58 months after achieving complete response. The authors suggest that in metastatic cases, "chemotherapy only delayed the recurrence of disease in both metastatic sites and in the primary tumor-bearing site" (38). Pritchard et al. (36) state that none of 35 patients with metastases at diagnosis survived 5 years (in comparison with the 19% survival at 5 years among 194 initially nonmetastatic patients).

The second group of patients (those who manifest metastases during or after primary treatment) invariably represents very diffi-

cult and frustrating problems in management. They are typical
of clinical situations now faced with increasing frequency in pediatric oncology where, in multimodal programs, the primary treatments are conducted with maximum intensity in efforts to achieve
cures. Thus almost always the effective drugs will have been utilized in multicycle combinations at high doses. Radiotherapy
will have been administered, where indicated, with curative intent.

Tumor recurrence may be noted in sites already exposed to
irradiation. Metastases may involve anatomic areas that may limit
the extent and degree of radiotherapy. Resistance to specific
drug(s) may be apparent or suspected. Although still effective,
the continued administration of a certain drug may be precluded
because of toxicity (such as hemorrhagic cystitis after CYT and
ADR-associated cardiomyopathy).

Since patients will differ with respect to fields and doses of
irradiation utilized in primary therapy and with respect to the
amounts and scheduling of drugs given previously, the planning
of postmetastatic therapy must be individualized. The strategies
usually required will include the following: (a) consideration of
reuse of a drug (or drugs) known to be effective but which had
been used before in the patient (there is the hope that the same
drug(s), particularly in a different dose/schedule combination
may provide some additional beneficial effect), (b) identification
of symptoms that require immediate palliative therapy (such as
severe bone pain or cord compression), (c) judicious utilization
of irradiation, (d) periodic determination of the extent of the
disease in the patient, (e) constant assessment of the balance
between anticipated benefit versus the discomfort and toxicity
of the treatment, (f) continual evaluation of patient so that ineffective regimens will not be prolonged beyond the period needed
for an adequate trial, and (g) periodic reorientation regarding
available therapeutic options, however uncertain the expected
result may be.

Published data thus far do not provide much encouragement
as to the long-term survival of patients who fail primary treatment
of Ewing's sarcoma. Reports of various clinical experiences create

the ominous impression that the ultimate prognosis is extremely grave, even though temporary good responses can be achieved by various drug combinations such as those already outlined above in primary therapy and new combinations such as ADR with dacarbazine (DTIC) (6).

Extraosseous Ewing's Sarcoma

Categorized as a tumor of specific type but of uncertain histogenesis (13), a pathologic entity described by Angervall and Enzinger (1) as "extraskeletal neoplasm resembling Ewing's sarcoma" has been recognized recently. This tumor arises in the soft tissues principally of the paravertebral region, chest wall, posterior mediastinum, and the lower extremities (1,13). This tumor occurs most commonly in late adolescence and early adulthood, affecting males and females equally. The tumor does not involve bone and must be differentiated from neuroblastoma, neuroepithelioma, synovial sarcoma, and particularly rhabdomyosarcoma (1,13,25,39).

Pathologically, the tumor consists of densely packed uniform round and oval cells. The cells contain distinctly outlined nuclei and scant pale staining cytoplasm. Intracellular glycogen can be readily demonstrated in all cases. The tumor would be called Ewing's sarcoma if it involved bone. Metastases occur chiefly to lungs and the skeletal system (1,25).

In the past few years, the Intergroup Rhabdomyosarcoma Study (IRS) has provided considerable material for histopathologic studies on tumors registered on study as rhabdomyosarcoma (29,39). In the initial review of 314 cases, 26 were considered to have "morphologic characteristics similar to Ewing's sarcoma of bone" (39). Two variants were noted. For convenience, one has been called "round cell type I." This corresponded to the conventional Ewing's sarcoma. The other was called "round cell type II" and corresponded to the "large cell" Ewing sarcoma (10).

These variants were more common in the older children in

the IRS, a collaborative pediatric investigation. With respect to the clinical status at entry into the study, eight of the 26 had had complete surgical resection, seven had microscopic residual disease, eight had gross residual disease, and three had metastases. None of the tumors involved bone as the primary site.

These patients were treated as rhabdomyosarcoma, utilizing the randomized treatment appropriate for the clinical grouping (29). Since there is a great deal of similarity in the basic approach in the programs for Ewing's sarcoma and rhabdomyosarcoma, therapy for the latter neoplasm would seem appropriate for extraskeletal Ewing's sarcoma. In the IRS, 17 of 26 have remained relapse-free 10 to 170 weeks (median, 113 weeks) at the time of the analysis (39).

Tumors of similar morphologic characteristics have been reported from time to time. Tefft et al. (44) described a paravertebral round-cell tumor in childhood which involved soft tissue but not bone. Close histologic resemblance to Ewing's sarcoma was noted. Recently, Askin et al. (2a) reported a similar round cell tumor of soft tissues about the thorax without osseous involvement. Glycogen, however, was not demonstrated in these cases. Whether or not all of these so-called extraskeletal or extraosseous Ewing sarcomas will be established as a pathologic entity, they do require, at this time, inclusion in the differential diagnosis of both soft tissue sarcomas and Ewing's sarcoma.

Second Malignant Neoplasms

The management of Ewing's sarcoma has been significantly dependent on the control of the primary lesion by high doses of radiation. The use of such irradiation in turn has been associated with the risk of a second malignant neoplasm (usually osteosarcoma) developing in the treatment field among the survivors (26,27,30,40).

In an attempt to estimate quantitatively the risk of radiation-related subsequent malignant tumors in survivors of Ewing's sarcoma, the clinical data were examined on 173 patients with this tumor treated at M. D. Anderson Hospital between 1944 and 1976 (40). From this group, 24 patients had survived without evidence of disease activity for 3 years or longer (3 to 22 years). Among these 24 patients, four new bone tumors (osteosarcoma) were observed in the heavily irradiated bones. One other patient developed malignant fibrous histiocytoma of soft tissues at 18 months in the irradiated area. This case, however, was not included in the calculations because the short latent period raised questions regarding cause and effect relationship.

The secondary osteosarcomas were noted after latent periods of 52, 74, 80, and 225 months, respectively. Among the 24 long-term survivors, the expected incidence of any new bone tumors was 1.2×10^{-3} cases. The risk associated with radiation after 3 years was 7.2 cases per million person rads per year. The cumulative cancer risk over 10 years among the irradiated long-term survivors was 35% (40). The rate of tumor development appeared to be most pronounced 5 to 9 years after diagnosis.

The extent to which the concomitant use of multidrug chemotherapy may have influenced the risk of second cancers is unknown. The relative rarity of Ewing's sarcoma and the small numbers of long-term survivors in most single institutional experiences have precluded detailed statistical studies of risks of radiation carcinogenesis. The absence of matched control populations further enhanced the difficulty of drawing valid conclusions.

In other tumors, such as Hodgkin's disease, it has been reported that there is a highly significant increase in incidence of new cancers among the intensively treated patients (2). This aspect needs considerably more study since published data suggest (at least statistically) that chemotherapy (AMD) may actually decrease the risk of radiation-induced second malignancies (12).

REFERENCES

1. Angervall, L., and Enzinger, F. M. (1975): Extraskeletal neoplasm resembling Ewing's sarcoma. *Cancer,* 36:240–251.
2. Arsenau, J. C., Canellos, G. P., Johnson, R., and DeVita, V. T., Jr. (1977):

Risk of new cancers in patients with Hodgkin's disease. *Cancer,* 40:1912–1916.

2a. Askin, F. B., Rosai, J., Sibley, R. K., Dehner, L. P., and McAlister, W. H. (1979): Malignant small cell tumor of the thoracolumbar region in childhood. A distinctive clinicopathologic entity of uncertain histogenesis. *Cancer,* 43:2438–2451.

3. Bacci, G., Campanacci, M., and Pagani, P. A. (1978): Adjuvant chemotherapy in the treatment of clinically localised Ewing's sarcoma. *J. Bone Joint Surg.,* 60(B):567–574.

4. Boyer, C. W., Jr., Brickner, T. J., Jr., and Perry, R. H. (1967): Ewing's sarcoma. Case against surgery. *Cancer,* 20:1602–1606.

5. Burgert, O., Gehan, E. A., and Nesbit, M. E. (1978): Prognostic factors in Ewing's sarcoma. *Proc. AACR ASCO,* 19:413.

6. Cangir, A., Morgan, S. K., Land, V. J., Pullen, J., Starling, K. A., and Nitschke, R. (1976): Combination chemotherapy with adriamycin (NSC-123127) and dimethyl triazeno imidazole carboxamide (DTIC) (NSC-45388) in children with metastatic solid tumors. *Med. Pediatr. Oncol.,* 2:183–190.

7. Chabora, B. McC., Rosen, G., Cham, W., D'Angio, G. J., and Tefft, M. (1976): Radiotherapy of Ewing's sarcoma. Local control with and without intensive chemotherapy. *Radiology,* 120:667–671.

8. Chan, R. C., Sutow, W. W., Lindberg, R. D., Samuels, M. L., Murray, J. A., and Johnston, D. A. (1979): Management and results of localized Ewing's sarcoma. *Cancer,* 43:1001–1006.

9. Coley, B. L., Higinbotham, N. L., and Bowden, L. (1960): Endothelioma of bone (Ewing's sarcoma). *Ann. Surg.,* 128:533–560.

10. Dahlin, D. C. (1967): *Bone Tumors. General Aspects and Data on 3,987 Cases,* second edition. Charles C Thomas, Springfield, Illinois.

11. Dahlin, D. C. (1978): *Bone Tumors. General Aspects and Data on 6,221 Cases,* third edition. Charles C Thomas, Springfield, Illinois.

12. D'Angio, G. J., Meadows, A., Miké, V., Harris, C., Evans, A., Jaffe, N., Newton, W., Schweisguth, O., Sutow, W., and Morris-Jones, P. (1976): Decreased risk of radiation-associated second malignant neoplasms in actinomycin-D-treated patients. *Cancer,* 37:1177–1185.

13. Enzinger, F. M. (1977): Recent developments in the classification of soft tissue sarcomas. In: *Management of Primary Bone and Soft Tissue Tumors,* pp. 219–234. Year Book Medical Publishers, Chicago.

14. Falk, S., and Alpert, M. (1965): The clinical and roentgen aspects of Ewing's sarcoma. *Am. J. Med. Sci.,* 250:492–508.

15. Falk, S., and Alpert, M. (1967): Five year survival of patients with Ewing's sarcoma. *Surg. Gynecol. Obstet.,* 124:319–324.

16. Fernandez, C. H., Lindberg, R. D., Sutow, W. W., and Samuels, M. L. (1974): Localized Ewing's sarcoma—treatment and results. *Cancer,* 34:143–148.

17. Fraumeni, J. F., Jr., and Glass, A. G. (1970): Rarity of Ewing's sarcoma among U.S. negro children. *Lancet,* 1:366–367.

18. Glass, A. G., and Fraumeni, J. F., Jr. (1970): Epidemiology of bone cancer in children. *J. Natl. Cancer Inst.,* 44:187–190.

19. Huvos, A. G. (1979): *Bone Tumors. Diagnosis, Treatment and Prognosis,* pp. 322–344. Saunders, Philadelphia.
20. Intergroup Ewing's Sarcoma Study (1978): Protocol for multimodal therapy for the management of primary, non-metastatic Ewing's sarcoma of bone, pelvic and sacral sites excluded. Activated November 1978.
21. Intergroup Ewing's Sarcoma Study (1978): Protocol for multimodal therapy for the management of primary, non-metastatic Ewing's sarcoma of pelvic and sacral bones. Activated November 1978.
22. Jaffe, N., Traggis, D., Sallan, S., and Cassady, J. R. (1976): Improved outlook for Ewing's sarcoma with combination chemotherapy (vincristine, actinomycin-D and cyclophosphamide) and radiation therapy. *Cancer,* 38:1925–1930.
23. Jensen, R. D., and Drake, R. M. (1970): Rarity of Ewing's tumour in negroes. *Lancet,* 1:777.
24. Johnson, R. E., and Pomeroy, T. C. (1975): Evaluation of therapeutic results in Ewing's sarcoma. *Am. J. Roentgenol. Radiat. Ther. Nucl. Med.,* 123:583–587.
25. Kissane, J. M., Askin, F. H., Nesbit, M., Vietti, T., Burgert, E. O., Jr., Cangir, A., Gehan, E. A., Perez, C. A., Pritchard, D. J., and Tefft, M. (1980): Sarcomas of bone in childhood. Pathologic aspects. *Natl. Cancer Inst. Monogr. (in press).*
26. Li, F. P. (1977): Second malignant tumors after cancer in childhood. *Cancer,* 40:1899–1902.
27. Li, F. P., Cassady, J. R., and Jaffe, N. (1975): Risk of second tumors in survivors of childhood cancer. *Cancer,* 35:1230–1235.
28. Linden, G., and Dunn, J. E. (1970): Ewing's sarcoma in negroes. *Lancet,* 1:1171.
29. Maurer, H. M., Moon, T., Donaldson, M., Fernandez, C., Gehan, E. A., Hammond, D., Hays, D. M., Lawrence, W., Jr., Newton, W., Jr., Ragab, A., Raney, B., Soule, E. H., Sutow, W. W., and Tefft, M. (1977): Preliminary results of the Intergroup Rhabdomyosarcoma Study (IRS). In: *Management of Primary Bone and Soft Tissue Tumors,* pp. 317–332. Year Book Medical Publishers, Chicago.
30. Meadows, A. T., Strong, L. C., Li, F. P., D'Angio, G. J., Schweisguth, O., Freeman, A., Jenkin, R. D., Morris-Jones, P. (1979): Bone sarcoma as second malignant neoplasm in children: Influence of radiation and predisposition. *Proc. AACR ASCO,* 20:126.
31. Nesbit, M. E. (1976): Ewing's sarcoma. *CA,* 26:174–180.
32. Nesbit, M. E., Perez, C. A., Tefft, M., Burgert, E. O., Vietti, T. J., Kissane, J., Pritchard, D., and Gehan, E. A. (1980): Multimodal therapy for the management of primary, non-metastatic Ewing's sarcoma of bone: An Intergroup Study. *Natl. Cancer Inst. Monogr. (in press).*
33. Perez, C. A., Razek, A., Tefft, M., Nesbit, M., Burgert, E. O., Jr., Kissane, J., Vietti, T., and Gehan, E. A. (1977): Analysis of local tumor control in Ewing's sarcoma. Preliminary results of a Cooperative Intergroup Study. *Cancer,* 40:2864–2873.

34. Pomeroy, T. C., and Johnson, R. E. (1975): Combined modality therapy of Ewing's sarcoma. *Cancer*, 35:36–47.
35. Pomeroy, T. C., and Johnson, R. E. (1975): Prognostic factors for survival in Ewing's sarcoma. *Am. J. Roentgenol. Radiat. Ther. Nucl. Med.*, 123:598–606.
36. Pritchard, D. J., Dahlin, D. C., Dauphine, R. T., Taylor, W. F., and Beabout, J. W. (1975): Ewing's sarcoma. A clinicopathological and statistical analysis of patients surviving five years or longer. *J. Bone Joint Surg.*, 57(A):10–16.
37. Rosen, G. (1976): Multidisciplinary management of Ewing's sarcoma. In: *Trends in Childhood Cancer*, edited by M. H. Donaldson and H. G. Seydel, pp. 89–106. Wiley, New York.
38. Rosen, G., Caparros, B., Mosende, C., McCormick, B., Huvos, A. G., and Marcove, R. C. (1978): Curability of Ewing's sarcoma and considerations for future therapeutic trials. *Cancer*, 41:888–899.
39. Soule, E. H., Newton, W., Jr., Moon, T. E., and Tefft, M. (1978): Extraskeletal Ewing's sarcoma. A preliminary review of 26 cases encountered in the Intergroup Rhabdomyosarcoma Study. *Cancer*, 42:259–264.
40. Strong, L. C., Herson, J., Osborne, B. M., and Sutow, W. W. (1979): Risk of radiation-related subsequent malignant tumors in survivors of Ewing's sarcoma. *J. Natl. Cancer Inst.*, 62:1401–1406.
41. Suit, H. D., Sutow, W. W., and Martin, R. G. (1977): Primary malignant tumors of the bone. In: *Clinical Pediatric Oncology*, second edition, edited by W. W. Sutow, T. J. Vietti, and D. J. Fernbach, pp. 605–635. C. V. Mosby, St. Louis.
42. Sutow, W. W. (1979): Chemotherapy of Ewing's sarcoma. *Prog. Pediatr. Hematol. Oncol.*, 2:97–106.
43. Tefft, M., Chabora, B. McC., and Rosen, G. (1977): Radiation in bone sarcoma. A re-evaluation in the era of intensive systemic chemotherapy. *Cancer*, 39:806–816.
44. Tefft, M., Vawter, G. F., and Mitus, A. (1969): Paravertebral "round cell" tumors in children. *Radiology*, 92:1501–1509.
45. Vietti, T. J., Gehan, E. A., Nesbit, M. E., Burgert, E. O., Pilepich, M., Tefft, M., Kissane, J., and Pritchard, D. (1980): Multimodal therapy in the treatment of metastatic Ewing's sarcoma. An Intergroup Study. *Natl. Cancer Inst. Monogr. (in press)*.
46. Williams, A. O. (1975): Tumors of childhood in Ibadan, Nigeria. *Cancer*, 36:370–378.
47. Young, J. L., Jr., and Miller, R. W. (1975): Incidence of malignant tumors in U.S. children. *J. Pediatr.*, 86:254–258.
48. Young, J. L., Jr., Heise, H. W., Silverberg, E., and Myers, M. H. (1978): Cancer incidence, survival and mortality for children under 15 years of age. *Am. Cancer Soc. Prof. Educ. Publ.*, 16 pp.

9

Osteosarcoma

The current clinical interests and significant investigative activities in osteosarcoma are related to therapy and may be listed as follows: (a) development of adjuvant chemotherapy regimens and evaluation of therapeutic efficacy of several programs; (b) modifications in drug administration (dose and schedule) to increase the intensity and effectiveness of different regimens e.g., use of weekly pulses of high-dose methotrexate (MTX) schedules and the preoperative administration of high-dose MTX pulses; (c) reevaluation of the usefulness of radiotherapy in combination with high-dose MTX; (d) development of techniques for limb-preservation approaches to osteosarcoma; and (e) aggressive treatment of metastatic osteosarcoma.

CLINICAL FEATURES

Osteosarcoma is the most common primary malignant tumor of bone, representing about 60% of bone cancers and about 5% of all malignant solid tumors in white children (80). Osteosarcoma constitutes almost all of the primary malignant bone tumors in black children, in whom Ewing's sarcoma is extremely rare (21). The clinical characteristics of osteosarcoma in children have not altered significantly in the past decades (see Table 1). Males are more frequently affected than females. If all ages are considered, 50 to 70% of the cases occur during the first two decades of life (up to 8% may be under the age of 10 years).

Femur is the bone most frequently involved as the primary site for osteosarcoma (40 to 50% of all patients), followed by tibia (about 20%) and humerus (10 to 15%). Less commonly involved are mandible and maxilla (7%), pelvis (7%), and fibula

TABLE 1. *Clinical features of osteosarcoma*

| | Source of data | | |
Parameter	Mayo Clinic (12)	M. D. Anderson Hospital (75)	Memorial Sloan-Kettering Cancer Center (39)
Study period	To 1976	1950–1974	1949–1974
No. of patients	962	243	210
Age range (years)	4–90	4–79	under 21
Males (%)	58.7	54.7	56.2
Age distribution (%)			
First decade	5	8	—
Second decade	47	61	—
Older decades	48	31	—
Primary site (%)			
Femur	42	50	53
Tibia	18	19	26
Humerus	10	11	16
Other	30	20	5

(4%). The region about the knee (distal femur and proximal tibia combined) accounts for 50 to 60% of all osteosarcoma. If older age groups are included, there appears to be relatively more frequent involvement of sites other than femur, tibia, and humerus.

CURRENT SURVIVAL STATISTICS

For decades, the overall survival rate among patients had remained consistently below 20% in practically all reported series (16). Treatment had consisted of surgical amputation generally but many with preoperative irradiation. After 1970, the survival statistics appear to have changed, with both the disease-free and the overall survival data showing significant improvement (see Tables 2 and 3).

Intensive and extensive use of adriamycin (ADR) (10,11) and

TABLE 2. Survey of published disease-free survival data

	Before 1970			After 1970		
Ref.	Chemotherapy	No. of patients	DFS[a] (%)	Chemotherapy	No. of patients	DFS %[b]
17,63,64	None	89	15	Multidrug	36	54
15,27,30	None	78	16	High-dose MTX	12	50
				High-dose MTX-ADR	22	73
36,39,51	None	210	21	Multidrug	31	69
9	—	—	—	ADR	88	39[c]

[a] DFS, disease-free survival.
[b] 2-year survival; [c] 5-year survival.

TABLE 3. *Overall survival in osteosarcoma:*
Current estimates

Ref.	No. of patients (N = 101)	Overall survival (%)[a]
17	36	79
39,51	31	77
15,30	34	80

[a] Mean, 78%.

high-dose MTX (25,30), as well as multidrug regimens (52,54, 60,61), began about 1970. Most published reports attribute the improvement in survival to the development of these effective adjuvant chemotherapy programs (15,17,39), although some are still unconvinced that chemotherapy has been responsible for the change (72,73).

The consistency with which improved results are being reported by various investigators and the magnitude of the differences in survival that have occurred are persuasive arguments for the value of adjuvant chemotherapy. Although comparisons were made with historic data and randomized studies were generally absent, it is ethically impossible to deliberately withhold at this time adjuvant chemotherapy from any patient with osteosarcoma. Moreover, there is no question that drugs and drug combinations have produced substantial tumor cell kill in osteosarcoma and have produced objective and measurable regression (even disappearance) of metastatic nodules for a substantial amount of time (11,25,29,52,69).

ADJUVANT CHEMOTHERAPY

The synthesis of the present adjuvant chemotherapy programs for osteosarcoma resulted from the following sequence of clinical activities: (a) demonstration of antitumor effect of new agents in patients with metastatic osteosarcoma; (b) careful evaluation of the pattern of toxicity of the new drug and assessment of potential use in combination with other drugs; (c) incorporation of the new drug into the program considered to be most effective at the time; and (d) clinical investigation of the new program with attention to adequate number of patients observed sufficiently long to allow valid conclusions.

The actual and progressive integration of various concepts and new therapeutic findings into adjuvant chemotherapy programs is exemplified by the review of the stepwise development of the regimens utilized by the Pediatric Department at M. D. Anderson Hospital (61) (see Table 4).

In 1962, osteosarcoma was considered to be an extremely chemoresistant tumor. At that time, first intimations that actinomycin D (AMD) was useful as an adjuvant agent in Wilms' tumor were being heard. The demonstration that phenylalanine mustard (PAM) could produce a marked regression of metastatic osteosarcoma in some patients, (57) initiated the efforts to develop an effective adjuvant chemotherapy program for nonmetastatic osteosarcoma (61,67).

By 1966, another chemotherapeutic concept, that of multidrug regimens in solid tumors, had been field tested and its effectiveness demonstrated in children with rhabdomyosarcoma (58). In an intensified schedule, the three-drug regimen of vincristine (VCR), AMD, and cyclophosphamide (VAC) was used in nonmetastatic osteosarcoma. The results indicated for the first time that survival rates in osteosarcoma might be influenced by effective chemotherapy (67).

Meanwhile, efforts were continued to evaluate patient tolerance to varying dosage schedules (66) and to examine new drugs for antitumor effect against osteosarcoma (69). Subsequently, major breakthroughs occurred when investigators of the Acute Leukemia Group B documented significant activity of ADR against osteosarcoma (11) and when Jaffe and colleagues (27) reported from Farber's service that massive dose MTX with citrovorum factor "rescue" (HD-MTX-CF) regimens caused regression of metastatic osteosarcoma. A multidrug adjuvant program combin-

TABLE 4. Systematic development of multidrug adjuvant chemotherapy for osteosarcoma[a]

Time period	Drug(s)	Refs.	Principle(s) tested and results obtained
1960–1971	PAM	57,66	Determination of antitumor activity of PAM used singly against osteosarcoma; antitumor activity (temporary) noted in 10% (2/19) to 43% (3/7) of patients with metastases.
1962–1968	PAM	66,67	Use as adjuvant chemotherapy in patients with nonmetastatic osteosarcoma; disease-free survival rate of 14% (2/14) achieved.
1969–1971	Pulse-VAC	58,67	Utilization of VAC regimen effective in another tumor (rhabdomyosarcoma) as adjuvant therapy in osteosarcoma; disease-free survival rate of 33% (4/12) achieved.
1970–1972	ADR	11	Evaluation of reported antitumor activity of ADR in metastatic osteosarcoma; antitumor activity (temporary) documented in about 40% (5/13) of patients with metastases.
1970–1975	CONPADRI-I	63,64,68	Adjuvant chemotherapy with four-drug combination (cyclophosphamide, VCR, PAM, and ADR); long-term disease-free rate of 55% (10/18) achieved; similar disease-free rate obtained in expanded SWOG Group study (24/44).
1972	High-dose MTX	25	Evaluation of reported antitumor activity in metastatic osteosarcoma of high-dose MTX with citrovorum factor; antitumor activity (temporary) reported in about 85% (6/7) of patients with metastases.
1973–1977	COMPADRI-II-IV	59,64,76,77	Addition of high-dose MTX to CONPADRI-I; extensive pharmacokinetic studies of high-dose MTX and development of systems for pharmacologic monitoring; intensification of high-dose MTX and ADR schedules to combat late metastases; long-term disease-free survival rate in COMPADRI-II-III (27/60) and (22/44) less than in CONPADRI-I; follow-up data from COMPADRI-IV still too early for analysis.
1977	COMPADRI-V		Intensification of high-dose MTX and ADR dose/schedule; "front-loading" concept; preoperative chemotherapy; "limb-salvage" surgical approaches; pilot studies well underway.

[a] Reproduced from ref. 61.

ing VAC with ADR (CONPADRI-I) was initiated in 1970 (61,68). Studies with a single agent adjuvant chemotherapy regimen with ADR were started in 1971 (9) and with high-dose MTX in 1972 (27).

The development of current adjuvant chemotherapy programs is exemplified by the COMPADRI-V regimen, which incorporates clinical and pharmacologic considerations that appeared to be significant in prior studies. The important features are: (a) intensification of HD-MTX-CF therapy by increasing the frequency (from triweekly to weekly schedule), dose (200 mg/kg or higher), and number of pulses; (b) intensification of ADR therapy by inreasing the total cumulative dose to 480 mg/M^2 for the program; (c) continued testing of the concept of "front loading," administering intensive therapy during the initial phases to achieve maximum tumor cell kill; (d) immediate chemotherapy with HD-MTX-CF, administering four courses preoperatively over a period of 4 to 7 weeks preceding definitive surgery; and

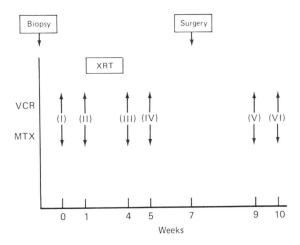

FIG. 1. Schema showing treatment plan for first 10 weeks of investigative regimen, COMPADRI-V. Numbers I through VI indicate pulses of VCR and high-dose MTX. Pulmonary irradiation (prophylactic) has been given during the interval between pulse II and pulse III of chemotherapy.

(e) provision of a therapy schedule that will permit the application of limb-salvage procedures at the time of definitive surgery.

Future modifications of the adjuvant program include the intensification of preoperative chemotherapy and the addition of prophylactic pulmonary irradiation. Several studies have indicated that high-dose MTX given on a weekly schedule is more effective than that given on a triweekly schedule (28,51). Prophylactic irradiation of the lungs is another reportedly effective measure (4) that can be added. Such irradiation can be accomplished in 10 fractions consuming a calendar time span of 2 weeks. This can be readily intercalcated into the chemotherapy schedule (see Fig. 1).

LIMB-PRESERVATION APPROACHES

The concept of local en bloc resection of bone tumor with prosthetic replacement is not new. For many years, homografts and allografts had been utilized in the treatment of giant cell tumors of bone and chrondrosarcoma (41,44,45). The demonstration that HD-MTX-CF therapy can cause significant tumor destruction of the primary tumor (24,53) has made the bone replacement approach feasible for patients with osteosarcoma (13,31,35,53).

The basic objectives of any orthopedic procedure for the management of bone cancer would include the following: (a) complete ablation of the tumor, (b) avoidance of amputation when possible, and (c) preservation of maximal function. The application of these precepts into the programs for en bloc resection and prosthetic replacement will identify the conditions and the patients most likely to yield successful results.

1. The patient (particularly those with lower extremity lesions) must have completed (or nearly so) the growth phase so that future increases in stature or length of extremity bones will be minimal.

2. The tumor must be resectable. Jaffe et al. (31) emphasize the important point that the tumor must be considered re-

sectable ab initio and that the chemotherapy "should not be instituted to render a suspected inoperable tumor operable."

3. Chemotherapy must be sufficiently effective to prevent further growth of the primary lesion. Effective chemotherapy will cause tumor shrinkage to facilitate surgery. Histologically, destruction of tumor cells will occur (24). When custom-made prosthesis is used, chemotherapy must control the tumor for the period of time needed (often 9 weeks or longer) to manufacture the prosthesis.

4. The patient must be free of demonstrable metastases.

5. Soft tissue involvement should be minimal so that satisfactory postoperative support for the prosthesis can be anticipated.

6. The patient must be psychologically prepared to accept amputation during the operative procedure if surgically indicated and any time subsequently if complications occur or the end result is unsatisfactory. The patient must also understand and be willing to accept the possibility of prolonged morbidity or of less than desired function of the part.

It seems obvious that additional clinical experience is needed to assess more precisely the criteria of suitability of the patient for the procedure, the nature of the best operative methodology, and the optimal preoperative and postoperative chemotherapy. Available data, however, clearly document the feasibility of this combined approach and the satisfactory results attained in many (13,31,35,53).

REEVALUATION OF RADIATION THERAPY

Over the years, the effectiveness of radiotherapy in the management of osteosarcoma has been viewed with fluctuating enthusiasm and disappointment. The possibility that irradiation can be used to sterilize the primary lesion has been investigated rather extensively (6). However, tumor doses of 8,000 to 14,000 rads given under conditions of local tissue anoxia failed to eradicate all viable tumor cells (56). According to published data from various sources, the overall survival rate among patients with osteosarcoma treated by radiation alone was 12.5% (18/143) at 5 years (16).

For a period of time, there was widespread acceptance of a program of initial irradiation of the primary tumor followed by delayed and selective amputation (7,34,70). The intent here was to control at least partially the primary lesion sufficiently long (several months) to select out for amputation the group of patients in whom distant metastases would be least likely to develop later. Among the objections to this approach have been the inadequacy to provide the anticipated palliation, the failure to demonstrate any improvement in survival rate, and the need, in many patients, to carry out emergency amputations under extenuating conditions for palliative reasons (3,32,33).

Recent results from the treatment of metastatic osteosarcoma provide a strong justification for the reevaluation of the role of radiation therapy in osteosarcoma. Clinical observations document significant regression of tumor for prolonged periods of time when radiation therapy is combined with high-dose MTX (25,52,62). The possibility that chemotherapy, such as high-dose MTX regimens, can enhance radiation effects justifies full investigation of the therapeutic potential of the combined modality programs in all aspects of treatment for osteosarcoma.

Reports from Japanese investigators suggest that fast neutron radiotherapy may be advantageous in controlling the primary osteosarcoma lesion (1,71). It is thought that fast neutron has a higher relative biologic effectiveness and a greater gain factor as compared with X-rays. Fast neutron radiotherapy has been utilized with promising results in a treatment program for functional preservation of the limb (22).

Bone Metastases

The combination of high-dose MTX and irradiation has proved to be effective in the palliative control of skeletal metastases in osteosarcoma (62). Following treatment with 2,000 rads in 5 days or 3,000 rads in 10 days, there has been consistent and prompt control of pain. Tumor growth ceases. The duration of control can be prolonged (up to 2 years), and it has been possible to perform successfully en bloc resection of the metastasis and prosthetic replacement of the bone. The therapeutic attitude is emerging that bone metastases should be treated intensively and persistently and that long-term control of the lesion can be a definite possibility.

Prophylactic Pulmonary Irradiation

In practically all metastatic cases of osteosarcoma, the lungs are involved, either alone or in combination with other sites (75). Because the lungs are the first site of spread in most metastatic cases, prophylactic irradiation at the time of primary surgery is a reasonable concept if effective radiation can be delivered. Unfortunately, the tolerance of normal lung tissues is limited, and the maximal tolerated dose (46) is far below the dose needed to damage the tumor cell. If massive doses of radiation do not eradicate the tumor elsewhere (3,6,32,56,78), the use of a small fraction of the needed dose to the lung nodules should be questioned. Data published recently, however, provide a different and meaningful perspective on the basic issue of prophylactic pulmonary irradiation.

Although earlier studies had produced negative results (42,48), the European investigators reported recently that, in a randomized, prospective study, 44 patients who received lung irradiation had significantly better survival (projected to be 43% at 5 years) than 42 patients without lung irradiation (projected 5-year survival of 28%) (4). No chemotherapy was given to these patients.

The concept of prophylactic irradiation of the lungs immediately following pretreatment with high-dose MTX is being tested at M. D. Anderson Hospital (62) (see Fig. 1). This approach is supported by anecdotal evidence that high-dose MTX courses followed by irradiation with 1,500 rads in 10 fractions can cause objective disappearance of small metastatic pulmonary nodules and partial regression of larger lesions. Pulmonary lesions have been controlled for periods up to 2 years by this technique. These observations, as well as those reported by others (25,52,78), suggest that radiotherapy effect can be enhanced when both high-dose MTX and irradiation are administered together.

On the other hand, the possible drug exacerbation of radiation effects on normal tissues must be kept in mind (52). Since the maximally tolerated dose is approached, the possibility of radiation-induced pulmonary damage is real (46). Even more important, many adjuvant chemotherapy regimens include significant cumulative doses of ADR. The risk of potentially enhanced cardiotoxic effects of the combination of ADR and cardiac irradiation must be accepted (20,38).

HISTOPATHOLOGIC CONSIDERATIONS

Histopathologically, Geschickter and Copeland (18) described two major categories of osteosarcoma: osteoblastic or sclerosing type and the osteolytic type. Dahlin and Unni (12) recently used the term "conventional osteosarcoma" to describe the majority of the osteosarcomas arising in normal bone. The conventional group was further subdivided, on the basis of the predominant histologic pattern, into osteoblastic (about 50%), chondroblastic (about 25%), and fibroblastic (about 25%) types. Separated out were osteosarcomas of other types: in jaw bones, in Paget's disease, in other benign conditions, postradiation, dedifferentiated chondrosarcoma, multicentric, malignant fibrous histiocytoma, telangiectatic, low-grade intraosseous, periosteal, and parosteal (12).

Although arbitrary, the classifications have permitted some degree of extrapolation to prognostic considerations. For example, osteosarcoma of the jaw bone and parosteal osteosarcoma (19,74) have considerably higher survival rates than conventional types. On the other hand, telangiectatic osteosarcoma is considered to possess high malignant potential with few survivors (37). The

Mayo Clinic investigators (12) have indicated that the osteoblastic and chondroblastic osteosarcomas were less favorable than the fibroblastic type.

Another approach to the evaluation of the prognostic significance of the histologic features is the assessment of the "degree of malignancy" of individual tumors. When the grade of malignancy was categorized numerically from grades I through IV (least to most malignant), grade IV lesions had significantly worse survival compared to those with lesser grades of malignancy (72).

The investigators at Memorial Sloan-Kettering Cancer Center have carried the histopathologic assessment one step farther; they have incorporated the concept of tumor sensitivity into therapeutic decisions (24,49). Based on studies of metastatic lesions after chemotherapy, Rosen and colleagues (24,51) have formulated criteria for histologic grading (grades I to IV) of the effect of chemotherapy on osteosarcoma. By applying these criteria to nonmetastatic patients receiving preoperative chemotherapy, Rosen et al. (24,49,51) have reported significant differences in disease-free intervals between grade III–IV responders and grade I–II responders.

Because of the changing concepts in the treatment of osteosarcoma, it would seem necessary to reexamine as precisely as possible the prognostic correlations among treatment, histopathology, and survival. It is possible (as exemplified by Wilms' tumor) that histopathology may be a significant determinant of response to treatment. Conversely, the changing treatment techniques may abruptly alter the expected biologic behavior of a given histopathologic type (see below).

SURVIVAL AFTER METASTASES

Less than a decade ago, survival after metastases in osteosarcoma was considered to be highly unlikely; the 2-year postmetastatic survival rates were reported to be from 2 to 6% (47,65) (see Table 5). After 1970, there was a significant improvement in postmetastatic 2-year survival rates to approximately 47%.

TABLE 5. *Postmetastatic survival in osteosarcoma*

Institution[a]	Refs.	No. of patients	2-Year postmetastatic survival(%)
Before 1970			
MDAH	47,65	62	6
MS-K	36,49	121	2
SFCC	29	62	6
After 1970			
MDAH	47,65	44	38
MS-K	40,49,55	14 operable	71
		31 inoperable	54
SFCC	28,29,79	39	[b]

[a] MDAH, M. D. Anderson Hospital; MS-K, Memorial Sloan-Kettering Cancer Center; SFCC, Sidney Farber Cancer Center.
[b] 16 of 39 disease-free 6+ to 65+ months.

Examination of the postmetastatic survival curves prior to 1970 indicates that 50% of the patients were dead within 3 months from time of metastases, and 90% were dead within 12 months (36). Therefore, 2-year postmetastatic survival rates exceeding 45% are an impressive improvement.

To determine what factors were significantly implicated in this change in prognosis after metastases, the survival patterns were determined in 106 patients with osteosarcoma in whom metastases developed during treatment in the Pediatric Department of M. D. Anderson Hospital from 1954 to 1975 (47,65). The patients were 20 years of age or less, had medullary osteosarcoma, and had demonstrable evidence of metastases.

Clinical characteristics that were evaluated as possible prognostic factors in postmetastatic survival included: age at diagnosis (under 10 years/over 10 years), sex (male/female), race (black/white/Latin American), site of primary (upper extremity/lower extremity/other), site of first metastasis (lung/bone/other), year of diagnosis (1970 or earlier/1971 or later), and time from diagnosis to metastasis (0 months/1 to 12 months/over 12 months) (47,65).

Statistical analysis indicated that only two of the various factors examined had a significant effect on postmetastatic time. One was the year of diagnosis. In the group of 62 patients in whom the initial diagnosis was made in 1970 or earlier, there were four survivors (6.5%). In contrast, there were 17 survivors (38.6%) among the 44 patients in whom the diagnosis was made in 1971 or later. The second factor was the length of interval between diagnosis and the occurrence of metastases. The poorest survival was noted among patients with metastases at diagnosis (1/19, 5.3%); the best was seen among those in whom metastases developed more than 1 year from diagnosis (7/14, 50%). In the patients in whom metastases developed within 1 year from diagnosis, 13 of 73 (17.8%) were living. No statistically significant difference was noted between those who had metastases at diagnosis and those who relapsed during the first year. All surviving patients in this study were living more than 2 years from time of metastases.

Additional analyses of these two factors demonstrated that the beneficial effect of delayed metastases was more evident in the group of patients diagnosed in 1971 or later compared to the group diagnosed in 1970 or earlier. In statistical terms, the "poor risk" patient (diagnosis in 1970 or earlier with metastasis at diagnosis) had more than 11 times the risk of death per unit time postmetastasis than a "good risk" patient (diagnosis after 1970 with metastasis 13 months or more after diagnosis) (47,65).

It is presumed that this improvement in survival times reflected the availability of more effective chemotherapy in recent years. The drug regimens with major therapeutic activity in osteosarcoma were developed in the 1970s: ADR (9–11,52,54), high-dose MTX with citrovorum factor (25,27,52,54), and *cis*-platinum (2,43).

The approaches utilized in the treatment of metastatic osteosarcoma have been elucidated from a number of institutions (14,

25,28,29,40,49,52,55,62,69,79). The therapeutic principles may be tabulated as follows: (a) aggressive and intensive utilization of multimodal approaches; (b) consideration and periodic reconsideration (when indicated) of surgical excision of metastatic lesions; (c) radiation therapy, postthoracotomy, of entire lungs with boost doses to residual or inoperable metastatic lesions; and (d) intensive multiagent chemotherapy (ADR, high-dose MTX, and *cis*-platinum) modified in individual cases, depending on the nature of premetastatic chemotherapy.

Late Metastases

Current chemotherapy regimens are capable of affecting significantly the osteosarcoma tumor cell population. It is conceivable, therefore, that the biologic behavior of the tumor (such as the time interval between diagnosis and recognition of metastases) may be significantly altered. If this happens, then the distinction between temporary disease control and cure becomes uncertain. For example, is chemotherapy simply delaying the appearance of metastases (5)? On the other hand, the deceleration in the rate of metastatic progression may result in altered expression of metastases so that the metastatic nodules may be fewer and isolated (26).

Studies of cases treated before 1970 provide background data for the temporal pattern of metastases that have occurred in patients with metastases. Marcove et al. (36) reviewed the Memorial Sloan-Kettering Cancer Center experience with 145 operative cases of osteosarcoma under the age of 21 years treated from 1949 through 1965. Of these, metastases developed in 121. Considering the metastatic cases only, 82 of the 121 (68%) had metastases within 12 months from diagnosis and 115 (95%) within 24 months from diagnosis. In another report, Taylor et al. (72,73) found from a statistical analysis of 362 cases of osteosarcoma treated at Mayo Clinic between 1963 and 1974 that practically all metastases were evident by the end of the third postoperative year.

Recent tabulations of patients receiving adjuvant chemotherapy indicate that late metastases continue to occur (59). Whether or not these late failures reflect the relative ineffectiveness of various treatment regimens and whether or not the frequency of late metastases will be greater than expected are important questions that need answers. It is obvious that follow-ups of disease-free intervals should exceed 4 years before conclusions can be drawn with acceptable confidence regarding the results of therapy.

CONSPECTUS

The approach to the management of the patient with osteosarcoma is now multimodal. The efficient and productive functioning of a multidisciplinary team requires collaboration and communication of the highest degree (see chapter on multimodal therapy). Furthermore, the proper motivation of any new program is fueled significantly only when successful progress is evident periodically. For this type of assessment of results to occur, the study plans must be structured systematically, and biostatistical support must be available.

Effective adjuvant chemotherapy regimens do not ordinarily emerge *de novo*. The evaluation of the feasibility of the concepts, the development of the tactical components, and the integration into an overall strategic plan require dedication, perseverance, flexibility, and, above all, time (50,61).

While the current data justify increasing optimism regarding disease-free control, survival after metastases, and limb-preservation among patients with osteosarcoma, cautionary attitudes must be maintained toward overenthusiastic statistical interpretation of clinical observations and the deleterious (early and late) effects of the treatment procedures. Investigations must be continued to eradicate the tumor, to prevent metastases, and to preserve functional limbs in greater numbers of patients. Other efforts must focus on more specific identification of the prognostic factors that determine outcome of treatment.

Although various immunotherapeutic approaches to osteosarcoma have been studied, there have not yet been any major breakthroughs. In a recent review (8), the investigations along these lines have been categorized into nonspecific agents, tumor vaccination, serotherapy, interferon therapy, leukophoresis, and transfer factor. Still another therapeutic concept periodically revived is the utilization of anticoagulants (23).

REFERENCES

1. Aoki, H. (1977): Studies of high-dose radiation therapy for osteosarcoma. *J. Jpn. Orthop. Assoc.,* 51:241–262.
2. Baum, E., Greenberg, L., Gaynon, P., Krivit, W., and Hammond, D. (1978): Use of cis-platinum diammine dichloride (CPDD) in osteogenic sarcoma (OS) in children. *Proc. AACR ASCO,* 19:385 (Abstr.).
3. Beck, J. C., Wara, W. M., Bovill, E. G., Jr., and Phillips, T. L. (1976): The role of radiation therapy in the treatment of osteosarcoma. *Radiology,* 120:163–165.
4. Breur, K., Cohen, P., Schweisguth, O., and Hart, A. H. (1978): Irradiation of the lungs as an adjuvant therapy in the treatment of osteosarcoma of the limbs. An E.O.R.T.C. randomized study. *Eur. J. Cancer,* 14:461–471.
5. Burchenal, J. H. (1974): A giant step forward—if. *N. Engl. J. Med.,* 291:1029–1031.
6. Caceres, E., and Zaharia, M. (1972): Massive preoperative radiation therapy in the treatment of osteogenic sarcoma. *Cancer,* 30:634–638.
7. Cade, S. (1955): Osteogenic sarcoma. A study based on 113 patients. *J. R. Coll. Surg. Edinburgh,* 1:79–111.
8. Camblin, J. G., and Enneking, W. F. (1979): Immunotherapy in osteosarcoma. In: *Bone Tumors in Children,* edited by N. Jaffe, pp. 215–231. PSG Publishing, Littleton, Massachusetts.
9. Cortes, E. P., Holland, J. F., and Glidewell, O. (1978): Amputation and adriamycin in primary osteosarcoma: A 5-year report. *Cancer Treat. Rep.,* 62:271–277.
10. Cortes, E. P., Holland, J. F., Wang, J. J., and Glidewell, O. (1975): Adriamycin (NSC-123127) in 87 patients with osteosarcoma. *Cancer Chemother. Rep.,* Part 3. 6:305–313.
11. Cortes, E. P., Holland, J. F., Wang, J. J., and Sinks, L. F. (1972): Doxorubicin in disseminated osteosarcoma. *JAMA,* 221:1132–1138.
12. Dahlin, D. C., and Unni, K. K. (1977): Osteosarcoma of bone and its important recognizable varieties. *Am. J. Surg. Pathol.,* 1:61–72.
13. Eilber, F. R., Morton, D. L., and Grant, T. T. (1979): En bloc resection and allograft replacement for osteosarcoma of the extremity. In: *Bone Tumors in Children,* edited by N. Jaffe, pp. 159–167. PSG Publishing, Littleton, Massachusetts.

14. Filler, R. M. (1979): Surgical treatment of pulmonary metastases from osteosarcoma. In: *Bone Tumors in Children,* edited by N. Jaffe, pp. 169–181. PSG Publishing, Littleton, Massachusetts.

15. Frei, E., III, Jaffe, N., Gero, M., Skipper, H., and Watts, H. (1978): Adjuvant chemotherapy of osteogenic sarcoma: Progress and perspective. *J. Natl. Cancer Inst.,* 60:3–10.

16. Friedman, M. A., and Carter, S. K. (1972): The therapy of osteogenic sarcoma: Current status and thoughts for the future. *J. Surg. Oncol.,* 4:482–510.

17. Gehan, E. A., Sutow, W. W., Uribe-Botero, G., Romsdahl, M., and Smith, T. L. (1978): Osteosarcoma. The M. D. Anderson experience, 1950–1974. In: *Immunotherapy of Cancer: Present Status of Trials in Man,* edited by W. D. Terry and D. Windhorst, pp. 271–282. Raven Press, New York.

18. Geschickter, C. F., and Copeland, M. M. (1949): *Tumors of Bone,* third edition. J. B. Lippincott, Philadelphia.

19. Geschickter, C. F., and Copeland, M. M. (1951): Parosteal osteoma of bone: A new entity. *Ann. Surg.,* 133:790–807.

20. Gilladoga, A. C., Manuel, C., Tan, C. T. C., Wollner, N., Sternberg, S. S., and Murphy, M. L. (1976): The cardiotoxicity of adriamycin and daunomycin in children. *Cancer,* 37:1070–1078.

21. Glass, A. G., and Fraumeni, J. F., Jr. (1970): Epidemiology of bone cancer in children. *J. Natl. Cancer Inst.,* 44:187–199.

22. Hodaka, E., Maruyama, K., Takada, N., and Tatezaki, S. (1979): Multimodal treatment including fast neutron radiotherapy for osteosarcoma. *Cancer Bull.,* 31:216–219.

23. Hoover, H. C., Ketcham, A. S., Millar, R. C., and Gralnick, H. R. (1978): Osteosarcoma. Improved survival with anticoagulation and amputation. *Cancer,* 41:2475–2480.

24. Huvos, A. G., Rosen, G., and Marcove, R. C. (1977): Primary osteogenic sarcoma. Pathologic aspects in 20 patients after treatment with chemotherapy, en bloc resection, and prosthetic bone replacement. *Arch. Pathol. Lab. Med.,* 101:14–18.

25. Jaffe, N., Farber, S., Traggis, D., Geiser, C., Kim, B. S., Das, L., Frauenberger, G., Djerassi, I., and Cassady, J. R. (1973): Favorable response of metastatic osteogenic sarcoma to pulse high-dose methotrexate with citrovorum rescue and radiation therapy. *Cancer,* 31:1367–1373.

26. Jaffe, N., Frei, E., III, Smith, E., Cassady, J. R., Filler, R. M., and Zelen, M. (1978): Hypothesis for the pattern of pulmonary metastases in osteogenic sarcoma. *Proc. AACR ASCO,* 19:400.

27. Jaffe, N., Frei, E., III, Traggis, D., and Bishop, Y. (1974): Adjuvant methotrexate and citrovorum-factor treatment of osteogenic sarcoma. *N. Engl. J. Med.,* 291:994–997.

28. Jaffe, N., Frei, E., III, Traggis, D., and Watts, H. (1977): Weekly high-dose methotrexate-citrovorum factor in osteogenic sarcoma. Presurgical treatment of primary tumor and of overt pulmonary metastases. *Cancer,* 39:45–50.

29. Jaffe, N., Traggis, D., Cassady, J. R., Filler, R. M., Watts, H., and Frei, E. (1976): Multidisciplinary treatment for macrometastatic osteogenic sarcoma. *Br. Med. J.,* 2:1039–1041.

30. Jaffe, N., Traggis, D., Cohen, D., Watts, H., Frei, E., III, and Cassady, J. R. (1979): The impact of high dose methotrexate on the current management of osteogenic sarcoma. *Medical Oncology, Research and Education,* 10:175–180.

31. Jaffe, N., Watts, H., Fellows, K. E., and Vawter, G. (1978): Local en bloc resection for limb preservation. *Cancer Treat. Rep.,* 62:217–223.

32. Jenkin, D. T. (1977): The treatment of osteosarcoma with radiation: Current indications. In: *Management of Primary Bone and Soft Tissue Tumors,* pp. 151–162. Year Book Medical Publishers, Chicago.

33. Jenkin, R. D. T., Allt, W. E. C., and Fitzpatrick, P. J. (1972): Osteosarcoma. An assessment of management with particular reference to primary irradiation and selective delayed amputation. *Cancer,* 30:393–400.

34. Lee, E. S., and MacKenzie, D. H. (1964): Osteosarcoma. A study of the value of preoperative megavoltage radiotherapy. *Br. J. Surg.,* 51:252–274.

35. Marcove, R. C. (1979): En bloc resection and prosthetic replacement in osteosarcoma. In: *Bone Tumors in Children,* edited by N. Jaffe, pp. 143–158. PSG Publishing, Littleton, Massachusetts.

36. Marcove, R. C., Miké, V., Hajek, J. V., Levin, A. G., and Hutter, R. V. P. (1970): Osteogenic sarcoma under the age of twenty-one. A review of one hundred and forty-five operative cases. *J. Bone Joint Surg.,* 52A:411–423.

37. Matsuno, T., Unni, K. K., McLeod, R. A., and Dahlin, D. C. (1976): Telangiectatic osteogenic sarcoma. *Cancer,* 38:2538–2547.

38. Merrill, J., Greco, F. A., Zimbler, H., Brereton, H. D., Lamberg, J. D., and Pomeroy, T. C. (1975): Adriamycin and radiation: Synergistic cardiotoxicity. *Ann. Intern. Med.,* 82:122–123.

39. Miké, V., and Marcove, R. C. (1978): Osteogenic sarcoma under the age of 21: Experience of Memorial Sloan-Kettering Cancer Center. In: *Immunotherapy of Cancer: Present Status of Trials in Man,* edited by W. D. Terry and D. Windhorst, pp. 283–292. Raven Press, New York.

40. Mosende, C., Gutierrez, M., Caparros, B., and Rosen, G. (1977): Combination chemotherapy with bleomycin, cyclophosphamide and dactinomycin for the treatment of osteogenic sarcoma. *Cancer,* 40:2779–2786.

41. Murray, J. A. (1977): The surgical management of primary neoplasia of bone. In: *Management of Primary Bone and Soft Tissue Tumors,* pp. 107–113. Year Book Medical Publishers, Chicago.

42. Newton, K. A. (1972): Prophylactic irradiation of the lung in bone sarcoma. In: *Bone—Certain Aspects of Neoplasia,* edited by C. H. G. Price and F. G. M. Ross, pp. 307–311. Butterworths, London.

43. Ochs, J. J., Freeman, A. I., Douglass, H. O., Jr., Higby, D. S., Mendell, E. R., and Sinks, L. F. (1978): Cis-Dichlorodiammine platinum (II) in advanced osteosarcoma. *Cancer Treat. Rep.,* 62:239–245.

44. Parrish, F. F. (1966): Treatment of bone tumors by total excision and replacement with massive autologous and homologous grafts. *J. Bone Joint Surg.,* 48A:968–990.

45. Parrish, F. F. (1977): Total resection of giant cell tumors of the extremities. In: *Management of Primary Bone and Soft Tissue Tumors,* pp. 115–119. Year Book Medical Publishers, Chicago.

46. Perez, C. A. (1977): Basic concepts and clinical implications of radiation therapy. In: *Clinical Pediatric Oncology,* second edition, edited by W. W. Sutow, T. J. Vietti, and D. J. Fernbach, pp. 139–181. C. V. Mosby, St. Louis.

47. Perez, C., Herson, J., Kimball, J. C., and Sutow, W. W. (1978): Prognosis after metastasis in osteosarcoma. *Cancer Clin. Trials,* 1:315–320.

48. Rab, G. T., Ivins, J. C., Childs, D. S., Jr., Cupps, R. E., and Pritchard, D. J. (1976): Elective whole lung irradiation in the treatment of osteogenic sarcoma. *Cancer,* 38:939–942.

49. Rosen, G., Huvos, A. G., Mosende, C., Beattie, E. J., Jr., Exelby, P. R., Capparos, B., and Marcove, R. C. (1978): Chemotherapy and thoracotomy for metastatic osteogenic sarcoma. A model for adjuvant chemotherapy and the rationale for the timing of thoracic surgery. *Cancer,* 41:841–849.

50. Rosen, G., and Jaffe, N. (1979): Chemotherapy of malignant spindle cell sarcomas of bone. In: *Bone Tumors in Children,* edited by N. Jaffe, pp. 107–130. PSG Publishing, Littleton, Massachusetts.

51. Rosen, G., Marcove, R. C., Capparos, B., Nirenberg, A., Kosloff, C., and Huvos, A. G. (1980): Primary osteogenic sarcoma: The rationale for preoperative chemotherapy and delayed surgery. *Natl. Cancer Inst. Monogr. (in press).*

52. Rosen, G., Tefft, M., Martinez, A., Cham, W., and Murphy, M. L. (1975): Combination chemotherapy and radiation therapy in the treatment of metastatic osteogenic sarcoma. *Cancer,* 35:622–630.

53. Rosen, G., Murphy, M. L., Huvos, A. G., Gutierrez, M. and Marcove, R. C. (1976): Chemotherapy, en bloc resection, and prosthetic bone replacement in the treatment of osteogenic sarcoma. *Cancer,* 37:1–11.

54. Rosen, G., Suwansirikul, S., Kwon, C., Tan, C., Wu, S. J., Beattie, E. J., Jr., and Murphy, M. L. (1974): High-dose methotrexate with citrovorum factor rescue and adriamycin in childhood osteogenic sarcoma. *Cancer,* 33:1151–1163.

55. Shah, A., Exelby, P. R., Rao, B., Marcove, R., Rosen, G., and Beattie, E. J., Jr. (1977): Thoracotomy as adjuvant to chemotherapy in metastatic osteogenic sarcoma. *J. Pediatr. Surg.,* 12:983–990.

56. Suit, H. D. (1965): Radiation therapy given under conditions of local tissue hypoxia for bone and soft tissue sarcoma. In: *Tumors of Bone and Soft Tissues,* pp. 143–163. Year Book Medical Publishers, Chicago.

57. Sullivan, M. P., Sutow, W. W., and Taylor, G. (1963): L-Phenylalanine mustard as a treatment for metastatic osteogenic sarcoma in children. *J. Pediatr.,* 63:227–237.

58. Sutow, W. W. (1969): Chemotherapeutic management of childhood rhabdo-myosarcoma. In: *Neoplasia in Childhood,* pp. 201–208. Year Book Medical Publishers, Chicago.
59. Sutow, W. W. (1976): Late metastases in osteosarcoma. *Lancet,* 1:856.
60. Sutow, W. W. (1975): Combination chemotherapy with adriamycin (NSC-123127) in primary treatment of osteogenic sarcoma. *Cancer Chemother. Rep.,* Part 3. 6:315–317.
61. Sutow, W. W. (1978): Primary adjuvant chemotherapy in osteosarcoma. *Cancer Bull.,* 30:178–181.
62. Sutow, W. W., and Chan, R. C. (1980): Irradiation and chemotherapy in pediatric tumors. In: *Textbook of Radiotherapy,* edited by G. H. Fletcher, third edition, pp. 637–661. Lea and Feibiger, Philadelphia.
63. Sutow, W. W., Gehan, E. A., Vietti, T. J., Frias, A. E., and Dyment, P. G. (1976): Multidrug chemotherapy in primary treatment of osteosarcoma. *J. Bone Joint Sur.,* 58A:629–633.
64. Sutow, W. W., Gehan, E. A., Dyment, P. G., Vietti, T., and Miale, T. (1978): Multidrug adjuvant chemotherapy for osteosarcoma: Interim report of the Southwest Oncology Group studies. *Cancer Treat. Rep.,* 62:265–269.
65. Sutow, W. W., Herson, J., and Perez, C. (1980): Survival after metastasis in osteosarcoma. *Natl. Cancer Inst. Monogr. (in press).*
66. Sutow, W. W., Sullivan, M. P., Wilbur, J. R., Vietti, T. J., Kaizer, H., and Nagamoto, A. (1971): L-Phenylalanine mustard (NSC-8806) administration in osteogenic sarcoma: An evaluation of dosage schedules. *Cancer Chemother. Rep.,* 55:151–157.
67. Sutow, W. W., Sullivan, M. P., Wilbur, J. R., and Cangir, A. (1975): Study of adjuvant chemotherapy in osteogenic sarcoma. *J. Clin. Pharmacol.,* 15:530–533.
68. Sutow, W. W., Sullivan, M. P., Fernbach, D. J., Cangir, A., and George, S. L. (1975): Adjuvant chemotherapy in primary treatment of osteogenic sarcoma. *Cancer,* 36:1598–1602.
69. Sutow, W. W., Vietti, T. J., Fernbach, D. J., Lane, D. M., Donaldson, M. H., and Lonsdale, D. (1971): Evaluation of chemotherapy in children with metastatic Ewing's sarcoma and osteogenic sarcoma. *Cancer Chemother. Rep.,* 55:67–78.
70. Sweetnam, R., Knowelden, J., and Seddon, H. (1971): Bone sarcoma: Treatment by irradiation, amputation, or a combination of the two. *Br. Med. J.,* 2:363–367.
71. Takada, N. (1976): Fast neutron therapy for malignant bone tumors. *Kanto J. Orthop.,* 7:65–72.
72. Taylor, W. F., Ivins, J. C., Dahlin, D. C., and Pritchard, D. J. (1978): Osteogenic sarcoma experience at the Mayo Clinic, 1963–1974. In: *Immunotherapy of Cancer: Present Status of Trials in Man,* edited by W. D. Terry and D. Windhorst, pp. 257–269. Raven Press, New York.
73. Taylor, W. F., Ivins, J. C., Dahlin, D. C., Edmonson, J. H., and Pritchard, D. J. (1978): Trends and variability in survival from osteosarcoma. *Mayo Clin. Proc.,* 53:695–700.

74. Unni, K. K., Dahlin, D. C., Beabout, J. W., and Ivins, J. C. (1976): Parosteal osteogenic sarcoma. *Cancer,* 37:2466–2475.
75. Uribe-Botero, G., Russell, W. O., Sutow, W. W., and Martin, R. G. (1977): Primary osteosarcoma of bone. A clinicopathologic investigation of 243 cases with necropsy studies in 54. *Am. J. Clin. Pathol.,* 67:427–435.
76. Wang, Y-M., Lantin, E., and Sutow, W. W. (1976): Methotrexate in blood, urine, and cerebrospinal fluid of children receiving high doses by infusion. *Clin. Chem.,* 22:1053–1056.
77. Wang, Y. M., Sutow, W. W., Sullivan, M. P., and Romsdahl, M. (1978): Preliminary studies of age and disease effect on the pharmacokinetics of methotrexate (MTX) following high dose methotrexate and citrovorum factor (HD-MTX-CF) therapy in children. *Proc. AACR ASCO,* 19:381 (Abstr.).
78. Weichselbaum, R. R., and Cassady, J. R. (1979): Radiation therapy in osteosarcoma. In: *Bone Tumors in Children,* edited by N. Jaffe, pp. 183–190. PSG Publishing, Littleton, Massachusetts.
79. Weishselbaum, R. R., Cassady, J. R., Jaffe, N., and Filler, R. M. (1977): Preliminary results of aggressive multimodality therapy for metastatic osteosarcoma. *Cancer,* 40:78–83.
80. Young, J. L., Jr., and Miller, R. W. (1975): Incidence of malignant tumors in U.S. children. *J. Pediatr.,* 86:254–258.

10

Cost of Survival

The durations of survival for most childhood cancers and the cure rates for many of them have improved significantly over the past 15 years. Concomitantly with these encouraging trends, however, it has become increasingly clear that the successes are exacting meaningful tolls. The cost of cure and the cost of survival must now be measured in terms of the nature, frequency, and severity of the deleterious effects that accompany cancer treatment (15,61,68). Aspects of the subject mentioned in this chapter include (a) types of late effects of therapy, (b) the problem of recurrence of tumor, (c) treatment-related oncogenesis, (d) possible genetic consequences of cure, (e) cost of cure, and (f) management of the patient who cannot be cured.

LATE EFFECTS OF THERAPY

Various investigators have published detailed inventories of the spectrum of late effects that have occurred at variable intervals from the completion of primary treatment (14,26,27,42,47,61). D'Angio (14) has classified the types of late adversities of treatment among long-term survivors of childhood cancer as follows:

A. Disruption of function
   1. Impaired growth and development
   2. Damage to central nervous system (psychologic, neurologic, and intellectual)
   3. Gonadal aberrations (reproductive, hormonal, genetic, and teratogenic)
   4. Disturbances of function in other organs and structures (liver, kidney, heart, lungs)

195

B. Oncogenesis
  1. Benign
  2. Malignant

Obviously, the frequency, severity, nature, and timing of the development of posttherapeutic disabilities depend on many factors, including location and size of the primary tumor, extent of the tumor, intensity of the local therapy, type of therapy, and physiologic status of the child. For example, impairment of renal function should not be totally unexpected in surviving children who had bilateral Wilms' tumor and received irradiation. Amputation is still indicated in most patients with osteosarcoma. Extensive local surgery is necessary in many patients with soft tissue sarcomas. Postoperative radiotherapy is included in multimodal management of residual tumor (microscopic or gross). In therapeutic doses, irradiation is injurious to normal tissues and posttreatment sequelae of various types developing immediately or later (even decades) should be anticipated (23,25,53,67).

An estimate of the incidence of clinically significant (moderate to severe) late effects has been provided by the Late Effects Study Group (47). In a multiinstitutional retrospective survey in 1979, the group investigated the sequelae of therapy in 369 survivors of childhood cancer in whom the diagnosis was established in 1972. The frequencies of significant sequelae of therapy among the children surviving the more common childhood solid tumors were: Wilms' tumors, 28% (15/54); soft tissue sarcomas, 54% (25/46); bone tumors, 81% (13/16); brain tumors, 53% (16/30); and neuroblastoma, 23% (7/31).

The nature of the deleterious effects of therapy also varied among the different tumors. In Table 1, the type and frequency of the late sequelae are compared between survivors of Wilms' tumor and soft tissue sarcoma.

Some adverse effects, particularly if lethal, are reported promptly in the medical literature. It is well-known that anthracycline antibiotics (for example, adriamycin) can cause dose-related cardiac changes ranging from electrocardiogram abnormalities,

TABLE 1. *Late sequelae of therapy*

Wilms' tumor (N = 54)	No.	Soft tissue sarcoma (N = 46)	No.
Splenectomy	4	Pelvic exenteration	7
Bowel resection/obstruction	3	Facial deformity	6
Impaired renal function	3	Severe sensory defect	5
Scoliosis, severe	3	Bony deformity	4
Amenorrhea	1	G-I disorders	4
Restrictive lung disease	1	Urinary tract disorders	3
Liver dysfunction	1	Soft tissue abnormality	3
		Severe growth failure	1
		Sterility	1
		Severe learning disability	1

a From Meadows et al. (47).

arrhythmias, cardiomyopathy, congestive heart failure, to death (38,52). Less well publicized is the risk of similar fatal cardiomyopathy that may follow cyclophosphamide therapy (51) and high-dose combination chemotherapy which included cyclophosphamide (3).

Most reported observations of the disabilities are based on clinical findings and probably underestimate the actual frequencies. Complicated or serial laboratory as well as extensive roentgenographic examinations are usually not included in a routine follow-up study (44). For example, the early diagnosis of secondary hypopituitarism due to a hypothalamic lesion after radiotherapy for nasopharyngeal cancer or primary hypopituitarism after irradiation of extracranial tumors will depend on a battery of laboratory tests of endocrine function (57). The development of clinical evidence of growth retardation and hypothyroidism may be a late manifestation. As the nature of the posttreatment complications becomes better identified and the etiologic circumstances more specifically defined, the risks as well as the significance of the undesirable consequences of therapy will be more precisely assessed.

LATE RECURRENCE OF TUMOR

While the problem of late sequelae of therapy is being determined in greater detail, both qualitatively and quantitatively, the total number of long-term survivors of childhood cancer is just now approaching magnitudes that may permit statistical estimates of the risk of late recurrence for specific tumors.

An approach in that direction has been documented by Li et al. (40). In a study of 140 Wilms' tumor patients who were surviving at 36 months, 14 subsequent late deaths (10%) were reported. In four patients, the tumor recurred; death in nine others was attributed to treatment-related disorders (including four from second malignant neoplasm arising in irradiated areas).

In Wilms' tumor patients, disease recurrence more than 3 years after treatment had been considered unlikely (10,11,29,37,54); but good data bearing on that question have not been published in recent years. Similarly, in patients with osteosarcoma, it had been generally accepted that the occurrence of metastases more than 18 months after amputation was extremely unusual (19). Recently, however, it has been reported (65,66) that late relapses have occurred 19 to 51 months after amputation in patients who received adjuvant chemotherapy.

These experiences underscore the need, in handling patients apparently cured of malignant solid tumors, to keep in mind the risk of late relapses. Of biologic importance, the phenomenon of late relapses generates questions regarding the true efficacy of some forms of adjuvant chemotherapy. The possibility that adjuvant chemotherapy in some patients simply delays the eventual development of metastases must be evaluated (8).

TREATMENT-RELATED ONCOGENESIS

The clinical enthusiasm over the achievement of successful control of several types of cancer in many children has been dampened significantly by the recognition that carcinogenesis may be a delayed consequence of therapy (22,41,45,46). Several etiologic possibilities may be considered: (a) the cancer therapy itself is oncogenic; (b) successful cancer therapy prolongs survival, providing the necessary period of time, for carcinogenic influences to act; (c) successful cancer therapy will prolong survival so that genetic tendencies (host susceptibility) for tumor development can become manifest; and (d) successful cancer therapy is now usually multimodal and multidrug. There may be synergism or interaction among the components of therapy that can increase oncogenic potential.

The problem of treatment-related oncogenesis necessitates the formulation of certain principles and attitudes among those who assume the responsibilities of providing cancer care:

1. The factors that may be related to oncogenesis in the surviving children must be studied and recognized.
2. The survivors who may be at increased risk of treatment-related oncogenesis must be identified (such as patients who have received radiotherapy, or genetically preconditioned retinoblastoma patients).
3. Treatment programs must be modified to reduce the number of treatment modalities to the minimum required for optimum results.
4. Optimum therapy must be defined in terms of both expected control rate and risk of second neoplasms.
5. The intensity of each mode of treatment must be reduced as much as possible (individual dose, cumulative dose, number of courses, duration of therapy).
6. Exposure to known environmental or occupational oncogenic factors (e.g., smoking or chemical carcinogens) should be minimized. There exists the possibility that the occurrence of the initial cancer represents an increased host susceptibility (common predisposition) to other cancers (6,22,62).
7. The relative oncogenic potential of specific anticancer agents should be determined so that a choice can be made among therapeutically similar agents.

8. Based on available information, follow-up studies should be structured to allow earliest possible diagnosis of any new tumors.

9. Under usual therapeutic circumstances, the risk of treatment-related oncogenesis is minimal (and acceptable) when compared to the risk of uncontrolled tumor progression if treatment is withheld.

The relationship between exposure to ionizing radiation and oncogenesis has been well established (24,50,55). Numerous examples of neoplastic development following therapeutic (17, 18,23,64) or accidental (12,43) irradiation have been published. Since radiotherapy involves high doses of radiation, the risk of carcinogenesis in the patient is substantial (39,41,45–48,64). There is the added factor that in very young patients, the risk of radiation carcinogenesis may be higher compared to older children (28). However, the extent to which age influences radiosensitivity needs further study (50).

From a life-table analysis of 410 patients living without relapse at 5 years after a diagnosis of cancer, Li (39,41) calculated a 12% cumulative probability of developing a new cancer in a 20-year interval. (The expected frequency of a new cancer in the general population of comparable ages was considered to be less than 1%.) When therapeutic irradiation has been used, the risk of new cancer increased to 17% (41).

Osteosarcoma appears to be the most common second malignant neoplasm in children who are surviving after treatment for a primary cancer (48). Based on a study of 24 survivors of Ewing's sarcoma from a patient population of 173, the development of new bone tumors (osteosarcoma) in four of the 24 was calculated to represent a cumulative cancer risk of 35% over 10 years for irradiated patients (64). Although the numbers of patients were small, the cumulative cancer risk was 70% over 10 years for patients treated with intensive multimodal therapy compared to 25% over 20 years for patients treated primarily by irradiation (64). When used, chemotherapy consisted of vincristine and cyclophosphamide in all patients with some receiving, in addition, actinomycin D and/or adriamycin. One report suggests that actinomycin D appeared to reduce the risk of radiation-related tumors (16).

Many of the major chemotherapeutic agents used in pediatric oncology are known to be potentially carcinogenic in laboratory animals (21,22,60,73). The drugs that bind tightly to DNA, such as actinomycin D, adriamycin, cyclophosphamide, and alkylating agents, are particularly carcinogenic (22,60).

The implication of chemotherapy in carcinogenesis in humans comes from case reports and retrospective epidemiologic studies. The increased occurrence of nonlymphomatous malignant tumors has been reported in patients with Hodgkin's disease treated with both intensive radiotherapy and intensive chemotherapy (4,7,9). Urinary bladder changes and neoplastic development reportedly have been associated with long-term cyclophosphamide therapy (2,13,28). Respiratory tract neoplasia has been linked to exposure to mustard gas (72). The excess occurrence of nonlymphocytic acute leukemia has been reported in patients with ovarian cancer treated with alkylating agents (56) and in multiple myeloma patients treated with melphalan or cyclophosphamide (34).

The degree to which the use of drugs in combinations and the concomitant administration of chemotherapy and radiotherapy enhance the hazard of carcinogenesis must be more precisely determined. Also unknown are the factors (e.g., immunosuppression) that determine the relative susceptibility of the individual cancer patient (20,58).

GENETIC CONSEQUENCES OF CURE

The child who is cured of cancer becomes an adult and in most cases can reproduce. Therefore, the assessment of the genetic consequences of cure and genetic counseling are important aspects of pediatric oncology (6,49,62,63). While the significance of the problem is recognized, documentation and accumulation of pertinent data are extremely difficult. At this writing, the potential genetic consequences are simply listed:

1. Both irradiation and cancer drugs may have cytocidal, clastogenic, and mutagenic effects on germ cells. Will such genetic damage to germ cells be transmitted to the offspring?
2. Family studies have shown a two- to fourfold increased risk of cancer of the same type in close relatives. The existence of "heritable" and "nonheritable" patterns of cancer has been recognized or suggested for some childhood solid tumors, such as retinoblastoma (30), Wilms' tumor (33), and neuroblastoma (31,32). Accordingly, there may be an increased risk of transmitting to the offspring an increased susceptibility for the same tumor.
3. Survival may subject the individual to increased risk with shortened latent period for the development of other cancers for which the individual is genetically predisposed (30).

COST OF CURE

Economic Cost

To the people who make up the family constellation for the child with cancer, the obvious and immediate consideration involves the financial cost (36). Current multimodal treatment for cancer requires intermittent, frequently prolonged hospitalization. The diagnostic procedures may be extensive, expensive, and recurrent. For adequate monitoring of ongoing and complex therapeutic regimens, regularly scheduled follow-up examinations and laboratory studies are necessary.

The financial burden for cancer care does not cease with completion of primary treatment. Even after apparent control of the tumor, long-term examinations are necessary to determine any late relapses of the cancer and, unfortunately, to detect and alleviate any therapy-related delayed side effects. The primary treatment process may be associated with unavoidable physical defects and dysfunctions that require active and prolonged rehabilitative care. Such treatments multiply the financial burden in both magnitude and duration.

Most families must face the ominous financial pressures fortified only with limited and/or dwindling financial resources. They must also accept the burden of related, nonmedical costs, such as travel and living expenses at the medical center while maintaining reasonably satisfactory economic conditions at home.

The difficulties in estimating the anticipated financial cost at any specific time during the course of treatment (but particularly at the beginning and during the phase of progressive disease) create uncertainties that plague the family. There can be a conflict between the desire to "have everything possible done" for the patient and the natural desire to "cut costs." The latter frequently takes the form of earlier discharges from the hospital and increased degree of treatments in the outpatient clinic and closer to home.

Psychosocial Cost of Cure

Medically, a child has cancer or has been cured of cancer, a discontinuum between disease-state and "cure" or "normalcy." Mental health, on the other hand, might better be viewed on a continuum scale from degrees of adjustment to degrees of maladjustment. The psychosocial impact of cancer on the patient, family, and society is receiving increasing study in recent years (5,35,59,68,70,74). Among the aspects considered in the assessment of life style and life quality among the survivors are (5, 68,69): disabilities (physical, behavioral and psychosocial); school performance and education; careers and employment; and marriage and parenthood.

The expression "quality of life" is now used with great frequency to denote an overall assessment of the interactions between an individual and society. While connotatively attractive, the term cannot be defined quantitatively. What is today's "normal" quality of life? How does one project this "normalcy" into the future?

Because the numbers of children cured of cancer are increasing, the psychosocial cost of survival is now being examined at (timely and significant) multidisciplinary conferences and workshops on subjects ranging from *The Normally Sick Child* (70), the *Care of the Child with Cancer* (1), *Status of Curability of Cancer* (71), to *The Truly Cured Child* (68).

THE CHILD WHO CANNOT BE CURED

Where the possibility exists that the treatment might cure the child with cancer, the physician is able to discuss readily with the patient and the family: (a) the statistical probability of cure, (b) the factors that may influence the outcome, (c) the nature, intensity, and duration of the anticipated treatment, (d) the risk of acute and late side effects, and (e) the quality of subsequent survival.

On the other hand, there will be a large number of patients (the percentages varying with the histopathology of the tumor and the existing clinical situation) where cure is not probable. What are the priorities, and how extensively and intensively should these children be treated? The management of such patients will require the structuring of new sets of values for therapy decisions. The complexities and the treatment of these patients will demand the best in the art of medical care.

Depending on the patient, the demands of the family constellation, and the depth of understanding among the people concerned, the physician may be subjected to unrelenting pressure of various types. Progressive spread of cancer can lead to breakdown of structural and physiologic systems in the patient. The child becomes increasingly symptomatic, and resistance disintegrates. The long-range perspective is clouded by the immediacy of various complaints. The cooperative family may become highly critical. Doubts and fears erode their previous confidence in the physician who is struggling under difficult conditions to maintain a reasonably comfortable existence for the patient. The physician may now be accused of callous disregard for the needs of the patient and disparaged for an inability to provide the depth and constancy of relief demanded for the symptoms.

The professional team in care of the child must anticipate the problems that accompany advancing disease. The family should be told frankly and early that the medical situation is unsatisfactory and that the deterioration may be rapid and symptomatic. This must be done without completely demoralizing the family. The family members are invited to participate with the physician in reappraising regularly the clinical situation and in adjusting the sense of values as conditions change. Careful discussions are held with the family outlining the objectives and capabilities of available palliative therapy. This requires careful maintenance of good communication and the assistance of all members of the team—physician, house staff, nurse, social worker, mental health professional, clergy, and others.

Pragmatically, conferences are utilized to discuss the causes of the symptoms and the available means for their alleviation. With respect to pain, the strategy and limitations of the administration of narcotics are explained, including such aspects as the anticipated dose and schedule changes, the use of combinations, the undesirable probability of addiction, and the eventual development of resistance.

On the positive side, the physician who handles children with cancer is obligated to keep fully informed of the ongoing clinical developments in the field of pediatric oncology that may result in changes in the treatment attitudes. One example is the increasing capacity to achieve apparent cures in children who have metastatic disease. This capability approaches 50% in Wilms' tumor patients, a magnitude of success not attained even in nonmetastatic cases of many other tumors. Importantly, successes of this type necessitate redefinition of frequently used expressions, such as "treatment failure" and "hopeless situation."

The second development is the possibility that even in seemingly hopeless situations, judiciously planned and executed multimodal interventions can provide the child with widespread cancer many years of meaningful life. The following case report will serve as an example of this type of attitude and the results that can be achieved.

> The patient, a 14-year-old schoolboy athlete, underwent left hip disarticulation in January 1974 for osteosarcoma of the left femur. Adjuvant chemotherapy was completed, at that time a 1-year program. In the meantime, the boy had attained new athletic skills in gymnastics, particularly with the rings. In September 1975, he developed swelling and pain involving the left radius. Biopsy showed metastatic osteosarcoma. With reluctance, an amputation was scheduled, but chest tomograms demonstrated lung lesions. The treatment plan was changed to high-dose methotrexate chemotherapy in conjunction with irradiation. By December 1975, he developed osseous metastases to the head and neck of the right femur (remaining lower extremity). Irradiation was expanded to include the right hip. There was good regression of tumor. In September 1976, left hip replacement was carried out with resection of the tumor. Two months later, the metastasis to the left radius was resected, and the wrist was stabilized using a prosthesis.
>
> Although chemotherapy was continued, pulmonary metastases recurred, and thoracotomies were performed in August 1977 and in October 1978 for resection of tumor nodules. Since that time, the patient, now a young man, has shown no evidence of tumor activity. The cost in terms of operative procedures, chemotherapy, and emotional stress was high; but the patient is alive 4½ years after the first metastasis. He has a reasonably functional left wrist, and he is ambulatory. He drives his own automobile. Most importantly, the disease appears to be controlled at this time.

Osteosarcoma, in the past, was a highly lethal disease. Prior to 1970, all but about 3% died within the first 12 months after the occurrence of metastases. With current aggressive multimodal therapy, 47% of the patients with metastases can anticipate long survival (66).

REFERENCES

1. American Cancer Society (1979): *Proceedings of the National Conference on the Care of the Child with Cancer.* American Cancer Society, New York.
2. Ansell, I. D., and Castro, J. E. (1975): Carcinoma of the bladder complicating cyclophosphamide therapy. *Br. J. Urol.,* 47:413–418.
3. Applebaum, F. R., Strauchen, J. A., Graw, R. G., Jr., Savage, D. D., Kent, K. M., Ferrans, V. J., and Herzig, G. P. (1976): Acute lethal carditis caused by high-dose combination chemotherapy. A unique clinical and pathological entity. *Lancet,* 1:58–62.
4. Arsenau, J. C., Sponzo, R. W., Levin, D. L., Schnipper, L. E., Bonner, H., Young, R. C., Canellos, G. P., Johnson, R. E., and DeVita, V. T.

(1972): Nonlymphomatous malignant tumors complicating Hodgkin's disease. Possible association with intensive therapy. *N. Engl. J. Med.,* 287:1119–1122.

5. Bartholome, W. G. (1979): The shadow of childhood cancer and society's responsibilities. In: *Proceedings of the National Conference on the Care of the Child with Cancer,* pp. 167–171. American Cancer Society, New York.

6. Bender, R. A., and Young, R. C. (1978): Effects of cancer treatment on individual and generational genetics. *Semin. Oncol.,* 5:47–56.

7. Brody, R. S., Schottenfeld, D., and Reid, A. (1977): Multiple primary cancer risk after therapy for Hodgkin's disease. *Cancer,* 40:1917–1926.

8. Burchenal, J. H. (1974): A giant step forward—if. *N. Engl. J. Med.,* 291:1029–1031.

9. Canellos, G. P., DeVita, V., Arsenau, J. C., Whang-Peng, J., and Johnson, R. E. (1975): Second malignancies complicating Hodgkin's disease in remission. *Lancet,* 1:947 949.

10. Cassady, J. R., Tefft, M., Filler, R. M., Jaffe, N., Paed, D., and Hellman, S. (1973): Considerations in the radiation therapy of Wilms' therapy. *Cancer,* 32:598–608.

11. Collins, V. P., Loeffler, R. K., and Tivey, H. (1956): Observations on growth rates of human tumors. *Am. J. Roentgenol. Radiat. Ther. Nucl. Med.,* 76:988–1000.

12. Conard, R. A., Rall, J. E., and Sutow, W. W. (1966): Thyroid nodules as a late sequelae of radioactive fallout—in a Marshall Island population exposed in 1954. *N. Engl. J. Med.,* 274:1392–1399.

13. Dale, G. A., and Smith, R. B. (1974): Transitional cell carcinoma of the bladder associated with cyclophosphamide. *J. Urol.,* 112:603–604.

14. D'Angio, G. J. (1978): Late adversities of treatment in long-term survivors of childhood cancer. In: *Proceedings of the Second National Conference on Human Values,* pp. 59–72. American Cancer Society, New York.

15. D'Angio, G. J., Clatworthy, H. W., Evans, A. E., Newton, W. A., Jr., and Tefft, M. (1978): Is the risk of morbidity and rare mortality worth the cure? *Cancer,* 41:373–380.

16. D'Angio, G. J., Meadows, A., Miké, V., Harris, C., Evans, A., Jaffe, N., Newton, W., Schweisguth, O., Sutow, W., and Morris-Jones, P. (1976): Decreased risk of radiation-associated second malignant neoplasms in actinomycin-D-treated patients. *Cancer,* 37:1177–1185.

17. DeGroot, L., and Paloyan, E. (1973): Thyroid carcinoma and radiation. A Chicago endemic. *JAMA,* 225:487–491.

18. Favus, M. J., Schneider, A. B., Stachura, M. E., Arnold, J. E., Ryo, U. Y., Pinsky, S. M., Colman, M., Arnold, M. J., and Frohman, L. A. (1976): Thyroid cancer occurring as a late consequence of head-and-neck irradiation. Evaluation of 1056 patients. *N. Engl. J. Med.,* 294:1019–1025.

19. Frei, E., III, Blum, R., and Jaffe, N. (1978): Sarcoma: Natural history and treatment. *Prog. Cancer Res. Ther.,* 6:245–255.

20. Harris, C. C. (1975): Immunosuppressive anticancer drugs in man: Their oncogenic potential. *Radiology,* 114:163–166.

21. Harris, C. C. (1976): The carcino-genicity of anticancer drugs: A hazard in man. *Cancer,* 37:1014–1023.
22. Harris, C. C. (1979): A delayed complication of cancer therapy—Cancer. *J. Natl. Cancer Inst.,* 63:275–277.
23. Hempelmann, L. H., Hall, W. J., Phillips, M., Cooper, R. A., and Ames, W. R. (1975): Neoplasms in persons treated with X-rays in infancy: Fourth survey in 20 years. *J. Natl. Cancer Inst.,* 55:519–530.
24. Hutchinson, G. B. (1976): Late neoplastic changes following medical irradiation. *Cancer,* 37:1102–1107.
25. International Commission on Radiological Protection (1966): The evaluation of risks from radiation. *Health Phys.,* 12:239–302.
26. Jaffe, N. (1976): Late side effects of treatment—skeletal, genetic, central nervous system, and oncogenic. *Pediatr. Clin. North Am.,* 23:233–244.
27. Jaffe, N. (1979): Pediatric cancer—delayed sequelae of cancer. In: *Proceedings of the National Conference on the Care of the Child with Cancer,* pp. 118–130. American Cancer Society, New York.
28. Johnson, W. W., and Meadows, D. C. (1971): Urinary-bladder fibrosis and telangiectasia associated with long-term cyclophosphamide therapy. *N. Engl. J. Med.,* 284:290–294.
29. Knox, W. E., and Pillers, E. M. K. (1958): Time of recurrence or cure of tumours in childhood. *Lancet,* 1:188–191.
30. Knudson, A. G., Jr. (1971): Mutation and cancer: A statistical study of retinoblastoma. *Proc. Natl. Acad. Sci. USA,* 68:820–823.
31. Knudson, A. G., Jr., and Meadows, A. T. (1976): Developmental genetics of neuroblastoma. *J. Natl. Cancer Inst.,* 57:675–682.
32. Knudson, A. G., Jr., and Strong, L. C. (1972): Mutation and cancer: Neuroblastoma and pheochromocytoma. *Am. J. Hum. Genet.,* 24:514–532.
33. Knudson, A. G., Jr., and Strong, L. C. (1972): Mutation and cancer: A model for Wilms' tumor of the kidney. *J. Natl. Cancer Inst.,* 48:313–324.
34. Kyle, R. A., Pierre, R. V., and Bayrd, E. D. (1970): Multiple myeloma and acute myelomonocytic leukemia. Report of four cases possibly related to melphalan. *N. Engl. J. Med.,* 283:1121–1125.
35. Lansky, S. B., and Cairns, N. U. (1979): The family of the child with cancer. In: *Proceedings of the National Conference on the Care of the Child with Cancer,* pp. 156–162. American Cancer Society, New York.
36. Lansky, S. B., Cairns, N. U., Clark, G. M., Lowman, J., Miller, L., and Trueworthy, R. (1979): Childhood cancer. Nonmedical costs of the illness. *Cancer,* 43:403–408.
37. Ledlie, E. M., Mynors, L. S., Draper, G. J., and Gorbach, P. D. (1970): Natural history and treatment of Wilms's tumour: An analysis of 335 cases occurring in England and Wales 1962–6. *Br. Med. J.,* 4:195–200.
38. Lenaz, L., and Page, J. A. (1976): Cardiotoxicity of adriamycin and related anthracyclines. *Cancer Treat. Rev.,* 3:111–120.
39. Li, F. P. (1977): Follow-up of survivors of childhood cancer. *Cancer,* 39:1776–1778.
40. Li, F. P., Bishop, Y., and Katsioules, C. (1975): Survival in Wilms' tumour. *Lancet,* 1:41–42.

41. Li, F. P., Cassady, J. R., and Jaffe, N. (1975): Risk of second tumors in survivors of childhood cancer. *Cancer,* 35:1230–1235.
42. Li, F. P., and Stone, R. (1976): Survivors of cancer in childhood. *Ann. Intern. Med.,* 84:551–553.
43. Mays, C. W. (1973): Cancer induction in man from internal radioactivity. *Health Phys.,* 25:585–592.
44. Meadows, A. T., and D'Angio, G. J. (1974): Late effects of cancer treatment: Methods and techniques for detection. *Semin. Oncol.,* 1:87–90.
45. Meadows, A. T., D'Angio, G. J., Evans, A. E., Harris, C. C., Miller, R. W., and Miké, V. (1975): Oncogenesis and other late effects of cancer treatment in children. *Radiology,* 114:175–180.
46. Meadows, A. T., D'Angio, G. J., Miké, V., Banfi, A., Harris, C., Jenkins, R. D. T., and Schwartz, A. (1977): Patterns of second malignant neoplasms in children. *Cancer,* 40:1903–1911.
47. Meadows, A. T., Krejmas, N. L., and Belasco, J. B. (1980): The medical cost of cure: Sequelae in survivors of childhood cancer. In: *Status of Curability of Childhood Cancers,* edited by J. Van Eys and M. P. Sullivan. Raven Press, New York *(in press).*
48. Meadows, A. T., Strong, L. C., Li, F. P., D'Angio, G. J., Schweisguth, O., Freeman, A., Jenkin, R. D., and Morris-Jones, P. (1979): Bone sarcoma as second malignant neoplasm in children: Influence of radiation and predisposition. *Proc. AACR ASCO,* 20:126.
49. Miller, R. C., Hill, R. B., Nichols, W. W., and Meadows, A. T. (1978): Acute and long-term cytogenetic effects of childhood cancer chemotherapy and radiotherapy. *Cancer Res.,* 38:3241–3246.
50. Mole, R. H. (1973): Late effects of radiation: Carcinogenesis. *Br. Med. Bull.,* 29:78–83.
51. Mills, B. A., and Roberts, R. W. (1979): Cyclophosphamide-induced cardiomyopathy. A report of two cases and review of the English literature. *Cancer,* 43:2223–2226.
52. Minow, R. A., Benjamin, R. S., Lee, E. T., and Gottlieb, J. A. (1977): Adriamycin cardiomyopathy—risk factors. *Cancer,* 39:1397–1402.
53. Perez, C. A. (1977): Basic concepts and clinical implications of radiation therapy. In: *Clinical Pediatric Oncology,* second edition, edited by W. W. Sutow, T. J. Vietti, and D. J. Feinbach, pp. 139–181. C. V. Mosby, St. Louis.
54. Platt, B. B., and Linden, G. (1964): Wilms's tumor—a comparison of 2 criteria for survival. *Cancer,* 17:1573–1578.
55. Radiation Carcinogenesis in Man (1964): In: *Report of the United Nations Scientific Committee on the Effects of Atomic Radiation.* Suppl. no. 14 (A/5814), pp. 81–110. United Nations, New York.
56. Reimer, R. K., Hoover, R., Fraumeni, J. F., Jr., and Young, R. C. (1977): Acute leukemia after alkylating-agent therapy of ovarian cancer. *N. Engl. J. Med.,* 297:177–181.
57. Samaan, N. A., Bakdash, M. M., Caderao, J. B., Cangir, A., Jesse, R. H., Jr., and Ballantyne, A. J. (1975): Hypopituitarism after external

irradiation: Evidence for both hypothalamic and pituitary origin. *Ann. Intern. Med.,* 83:771–777.

58. Schein, P. S., and Winokur, S. H. (1975): Immunosuppressive and cytotoxic chemotherapy: Long-term complications. *Ann. Intern. Med.,* 82:84–95.

59. Schulman, J. L., and Kupst, M. J. (1979): The emotional impact of childhood cancer on the patient. In: *Proceedings of the National Conference on the Care of the Child with Cancer,* pp. 144–149. American Cancer Society, New York.

60. Sieber, S. M., and Adamson, R. H. (1975): Toxicity of antineoplastic agents in man: Chromosomal aberrations, antifertility effects, congenital malformations and carcinogenic potential. *Adv. Cancer Res.,* 22:57–155.

61. Simone, J. V., Aur, R. J. A., Hustu, H. O., Verzosa, M. S., and Pinkel, D. (1978): Three to ten years after cessation of therapy in children with leukemia. *Cancer,* 42:839–844.

62. Strong, L. C. (1977): Genetic considerations in pediatric oncology. In: *Clinical Pediatric Oncology,* second edition, edited by W. W. Sutow, T. J. Vietti, and D. J. Fernbach, pp. 16–32. C. V. Mosby, St. Louis.

63. Strong, L. C. (1978): Genetic considerations. In: *Proceedings of the Second National Conference on Human Values,* pp. 210–219. American Cancer Society, New York.

64. Strong, L. C., Herson, J., Osborne, B. M., and Sutow, W. W. (1979): Risk of radiation-related subsequent malignant tumors in survivors of Ewing's sarcoma. *J. Natl. Cancer Inst.,* 62:1401–1406.

65. Sutow, W. W. (1976): Late metastases in osteosarcoma. *Lancet,* 1:856.

66. Sutow, W. W., Herson, J., and Perez, C. (1980): Survival after metastasis in osteosarcoma. *Natl. Cancer Inst. Monogr. (in press).*

67. Upton, A. C. (1968): Effects of radiation on man. *Ann. Rev. Nucl. Sci.,* 18:495–528.

68. van Eys, J. (editor) (1977): *The Truly Cured Child.* University Park Press, Baltimore.

69. van Eys, J. (1977): The outlook for the child with cancer. *J. Public Health,* 47:165–169.

70. van Eys, J. (editor) (1979): *The Normally Sick Child.* University Park Press, Baltimore.

71. van Eys, J., and Sullivan, M. P. (editors) (1980): *Status of Curability of Childhood Cancers.* Raven Press, New York *(in press).*

72. Wada, S., Miyanishi, M., Nishimoto, Y., Kambe, S., and Miller, R. W. (1968): Mustard gas as a cause of respiratory neoplasia in man. *Lancet,* 2:1161–1163.

73. Weisburger, E. K. (1977): Bioassay program for carcinogenic hazards of cancer chemotherapeutic agents. *Cancer,* 40:1935–1949.

74. Zwartjes, W. J. (1979): Education of the child with cancer. In: *Proceedings of the National Conference on the Care of the Child with Cancer,* pp. 150–155. American Cancer Society, New York.

11

Epilogue

Pediatric oncology is establishing an impressive track record at the forefront of medicine's onslaught against cancer. Many of today's effective management programs were conceptually structured, field tested, and first utilized in the treatment of childhood malignant tumors. Aspects of the activities responsible in major ways for the current attitudes in pediatric oncology have been mentioned in different parts of this book. Such discussions are limited by existing inadequacies of both knowledge and clinical capabilities.

Listed below for emphasis are some of the principles and approaches that have contributed significantly to the improving prognosis in children with malignant solid tumors.

BETTER KNOWLEDGE OF ETIOLOGY AND GENETICS

The interactions of genetic and etiologic factors are assuming increasing importance in the understanding and management of childhood cancers. The basic objective is the assessment of the risk of cancer in a given child. Thus approached, the practice of preventive oncology becomes a viable concept.

If the susceptible populations are identified (2,5) and the environmental oncogenic agents known, protective measures of varying intensity and complexity can be instituted, ultimately for the prevention of oncogenesis but more immediately for the prevention of cancer deaths. The measures, therefore, may include screening techniques for the early diagnosis and search for preneoplastic lesions. A further strategy would be the use of prophylactic extirpative surgery of the target organs. At this time, the most obvious situations where this approach might be considered include several familial cancers (4), such as colon, breast, and ovarian cancer. Elective colectomy, mastectomy, and ovariectomy are all surgical measures that can be readily carried out if the indications are acceptable. Ethical, social, and psychologic considerations may surface, but the estimation of the magnitudes of the risk of cancer should carry the greatest weight in reaching therapeutic decisions.

The risk of cancer is increased in a number of genetic syndromes. Examples include breast cancer in males with Klinefelter's syndrome, gonadal malignancy in gonadal dysgenesis, possibly testicular cancer in cryptorchidism, and ectodermal malignancies in von Recklinghausen's disease.

IDENTIFICATION OF PROGNOSTIC FACTORS

A major development in clinical pediatric oncology has been the more precise determination of the statistical correlation between the outcome of therapy (survival) and the presence or absence of certain pretreatment characteristics. Systematic studies of increased numbers of patients, along with improvement in survival, have established the value of these factors in predicting eventual outcome (measured as cure rate, duration of survival, length of disease-free state). Well-known examples are stage and age, as well as skeletal metastases in neuroblastoma, histopathology and stage in Wilms' tumor, and stage and site of primary lesions in rhabdomyosarcoma.

Of even greater significance is the current utilization of these prognostic factors in making therapeutic decisions. Thus in patients with favorable factors, the possibility of refining therapy (using less intense programs) is being explored. Patients with unfavorable prognostic factors are treated with more aggressive approaches. Specific examples include the documentation of the effectiveness of less intensive therapy in certain patients with Wilms' tumor (omission of postoperative radiotherapy to tumor beds and shortened duration of chemotherapy) and rhabdomyosarcoma (omission of postoperative radiotherapy and change from three- to two-drug chemotherapy). Where unfavorable prognostic features exist, therapy has been intensified (such as in patients with Wilms' tumor of unfavorable histology and in children with parameningeal rhabdomyosarcoma).

DEFINITION OF OBJECTIVES OF THERAPY

The prerequisite for the implementation of any therapeutic program is the definition of the general objective. To attain the objective, the physician requires first-hand evaluation of the available means and a concept of the probability of success. Such knowledge is essential not only in planning the details of treatment but especially in communicating with the patient and the family. Data have been compiled in various chapters of this book to provide basic information regarding these aspects. The objectives of therapy can be outlined as follows: (a) cure, (b) long-term, meaningful palliation, (c) rehabilitation, (d) temporary symptomatic palliation, (e) prevention, and (f) clinical investigation.

STRATEGY AND TACTICS OF THERAPY

The general principles of therapy are examined in detail in the chapter dealing with the child with cancer and especially in the chapter on multimodal therapy. The application of these principles to specific clinical situations is discussed in the tumor-oriented chapters.

SALVAGE OF METASTATIC DISEASE

By definition, all malignant solid neoplasms can metastasize. For patients who have received or are receiving primary treatment for the tumor, the development of metastases signifies ineffectiveness of or resistance to the treatment regimen. When metastases are present at diagnosis, they may represent rapid tumor growth and/or delay in diagnosis.

Until recently, clinicians were prone to approach the treatment of metastases with a defeatist attitude. Now, with the availability of more effective and intensive multimodal therapy, it is possible to provide meaningful although temporary palliation in most patients and, depending on the tumor type, to achieve long-term control in increasing numbers. Notable examples are Wilms' tumor and osteosarcoma.

The impact of premetastatic therapy on postmetastatic approaches and the possibility of induced alterations in the biologic behavior of the tumors are other cogent reasons to derive a general perspective of the problems of treating metastases. The prognostic aspects of the treatments are included in discussions of specific tumors. For each tumor, the clinician should be aware of certain basic information:

A. The magnitude of the problem
   1. How many are metastatic at diagnosis?
   2. How many can be expected to develop metastases during or after treatment?
   3. What is the risk of late metastases?
   4. What is the "salvage" or "retrieval" rate with best current treatment?

B. Biologic considerations
   1. What are the sites of predilection of metastases?
   2. How rapidly does the tumor progress?
   3. Do metastases follow some predictable sequence?
   4. What is the usual pattern of metastases (single, multiple)?
   5. Are there known premetastatic factors of prognostic significance for estimation of postmetastatic survival? (Examples are relation of "favorable histology" to better postmetastatic survival in Wilms' tumor, the correlation of delayed "time to metastases" with better survival in metastatic osteosarcoma, and the favorable influence of very young age in survival of children with widespread neuroblastoma.)

6. Do cell kinetic characteristics and growth rate patterns of solid tumors (7–10) provide any leads to treatment designs and to potential responsiveness to such therapy?

C. Clinical considerations
   1. How can diagnostic precision be improved to detect metastases earlier?
   2. What prophylactic measures can be applied? (Examples are regional lymph node dissection as part of primary therapy and prophylactic radiotherapy in parameningeal rhabdomyosarcoma.)
   3. What is the effectiveness (and morbidity) of adjuvant therapy (both chemotherapy and radiotherapy) in the eradication of occult metastases?

CURE OF CANCER

In the foregoing chapters on general considerations, the child with cancer, and cost of survival, various aspects of the concept of cure are examined. The implications of the concept are multifaceted, involving clinical, biologic, functional, and emotional parameters (3,6). They demand careful and constant study by the oncologist and the management team. Many years ago, Farber (1) epitomized the entire therapeutic approach to the child with cancer as "total care." Today, the overall perspective may well be broadened to the concept of "total cure."

RECENT REFERENCES

The preparation of the manuscripts and publication require considerable time, in the case of this book a period exceeding 2 years. During that interim, a continuous array of important papers has been published in a plethora of medical journals. It is an impossible task to keep satisfactorily abreast of all significant publications, even with the help of title listings, such as the *Index Medicus, Current Contents, Cancergrams,* and local/regional library circulars. As this book goes to press, there has been appended at the end of the bibliography section for this chapter, a list of references which were unavoidably omitted and which were thought to be appropriate for the various chapters.

REFERENCES

1. Farber, S. (1969): The control of cancer in children. In: *Neoplasia in Childhood,* pp. 321–327. Yearbook Medical Publishers, Chicago.
2. Fraumeni, J. F., Jr. (editor) (1975): *Persons at High Risk of Cancer. An Approach to Cancer Etiology and Control.* Academic, New York.
3. Frei, E., III, and Gehan, E. A. (1971): Definition of cure for Hodgkin's disease. *Cancer Res.,* 31:1828–1833.
4. Lynch, H. T., Guirgis, H. A., Lynch, P. M., Lynch, J. F., and Harris, R. E. (1977): Familial cancer syndromes: A survey. *Cancer,* 39:1862–1881.
5. Mulvihill, J. J. (1975): Congential and genetic disease. *Persons at High Risk of Cancer. An Approach to Cancer Etiology and Control,* edited by J. F. Fraumeni, Jr., pp. 3–35. Academic, New York.
6. Pinkel, D. (1979): Cure of the child with cancer definition and prospective. In: *Proceedings of the National Conference on the Care of the Child With Cancer,* pp. 191–200. American Cancer Society, New York.
7. Schabel, F. M., Jr. (1969): The use of tumor growth kinetics in planning "curative" chemotherapy of advanced solid tumors. *Cancer Res.,* 29:2384–2389.
8. Shackney, S. E., McCormack, G. W., and Cuchural, G. J., Jr. (1978): Growth rate patterns of solid tumors and their retation to responsiveness to therapy. *Ann. Int. Med.,* 89:107–121.
9. Skipper, H. E., Schabel, F. M., Jr., Mellett, L. B., Montgomery, J. A., Wilkoff, L. J., Lloyd, H. H., and Brockman, W. (1970): Implications of biochemical, cytokinetic, pharmacologic, and toxicologic relationships in the design of optimum therapeutic schedules. *Cancer Chemother. Rep.,* 54:431–450.
10. Valeriote, F., and Vietti, T. J. (1977): Cellular kinetics and conceptual basis of chemotherapy. In: *Clinical Pediatric Oncology,* second edition, edited by W. W. Sutow, T. J. Vietti, and D. J. Fernbach, pp. 182–196. C. V. Mosby, St. Louis.

RECENT REFERENCES

General Aspects

Cohen, A. J., Li, F. P., Berg, S., Marchetto, D. J., Tsai, S., Jacobs, S. C., and Brown, R. S. (1979): Hereditary renal-cell carcinoma associated with a chromosomal translocation. *N. Engl. J. Med.,* 301:592–595.

Greenberg, D. M. (1980): The case against Laetrile. The fraudulent cancer remedy. *Cancer,* 45:799–807.

Higginson, J., and Muir, C. S. (1979): Environmental carcinogenesis: Misconceptions and limitations to cancer control. *J. Natl. Cancer Inst.,* 63:1291–1298.

Janssen, W. F. (1979): Cancer quackery—the past in the present. *Semin. Oncol.,* 6:526–536.

Kennedy, B. J., and Lillehaugen, A. (1979): Patient recall of informed consent. *Med. Pediatr. Oncol.,* 7:173–178.

Li, F. P., Fine, W., Jaffe, N., Holmes, G. E., and Holmes, F. F. (1979): Offspring of patients treated for cancer in childhood. *J. Natl. Cancer Inst.,* 62:1193–1197.

Lynch, H. T., Follett, K. L., Lynch, P. M., Albano, W. A., Mailliard, J. L., Pierson, M. L. (1979): Family history in an oncology clinic. Implications for cancer genetics. *JAMA,* 242:1268–1272.

Staquet, M. J., Rozencweig, M., Von Hoff, D. D., and Muggia, F. M. (1979): The delta and epsilon errors in the assessment of cancer clinical trials. *Cancer Treat. Rep.,* 63:1917–1921.

Multimodal Approach

Conference on combined modalities. (1979): Chemotherapy/radiotherapy. *Int. J. Radiat. Oncol. Biol. Phys.,* 5:1425–1723.

Conference on combined modalities. (1979): Chemotherapy/radiotherapy (part 1). *Int. J. Radiat. Oncol. Biol. Phys.,* 5:1139–1423.

Jaffe, N., Filer, R. M., Cassady, J. R., Watts, H., and Vawter, G. F. (1978): Integrated multidisciplinary treatment for pediatric solid tumors. In: *Cancer—A Manual for Practitioners,* fifth edition, pp. 279–288. American Cancer Society, Massachusetts Division, Boston.

Chemotherapy

Al-Sarraf, M., and Baker, L. H. (1979): Transfer factor. *Cancer Treat. Rev.,* 6:209–215.

Gutierrez, M. L., and Crooke, S. T. (1979): Pediatric cancer chemotherapy: An updated review I. cis-Diamminedichloroplatinum II (cisplatin) VM-26 (teniposide), VP-16 (etoposide), mitomycin C. *Cancer Treat. Rev.,* 6:153–164.

Priestman, T. J. (1979): Interferon: An anti-cancer agent? *Cancer Treat. Rev.* 6:223–237.

Proceedings of the National Cancer Institute Conference on cis-Platinum and Testicular Cancer. (1975). *Cancer Treat. Rep.,* 63:1431–1695.

Skipper, H. F. (1979): Historic milestones in cancer biology: A few that are important in cancer treatment (revisited). *Semin. Oncol.,* 6:506–514.

Vietti, T. J., Nitschke, R., Starling, K. A., and van Eys, J. (1979): Evaluation of cis-dichlorodiammineplatinum (II) in children with malignant disease: Southwest Oncology Group Studies. *Cancer Treat. Rep.,* 63:1611–1614.

Zubrod, C. G. (1979): Historic milestones in curative chemotherapy. *Semin. Oncol.,* 6:490–505.

Neuroblastoma

Elkon, D., Hightower, S. I., Lim, M. L., Cantrell, R. W., and Constable, W. C. (1979): Esthesioneuroblastoma. *Cancer,* 44:1087–1094.

Evans, A. E., Chatten, J., D'Angio, G. J., Gerson, J. M., Robinson, J., and Schnaufer, L. (1980): A review of 17 IV-S neuroblastoma patients at the Children's Hospital of Philadelphia. *Cancer,* 45:833–839.

Finkelstein, J. Z., Klemperer, M. R., Evans, A., Bernstein, I., Leikin, S., McCreadie, S., Grosfeld, J., Hittle, R., Weiner, J., Sather, H., and Hammond, D. (1979): Multiagent chemotherapy for children with metastatic neuroblastoma: A report from Children's Cancer Study Group. *Med. Pediatr. Oncol.,* 6:179–188.

Lopez, R., Karakonsis, C., and Rao, U. (1980): Treatment of adult neuroblastoma. *Cancer,* 45:840–844.

Wilms' Tumor

Lennox, E. L., Stiller, C. A., Morris Jones, P. H., and Kinnier-Wilson, L. M. (1979): Nephroblastoma: Treatment during 1970–3 and the effect on survival of inclusion in the first MRC trials. *Br. Med. J.,* 2:567–569.

Martin, L. W., Schaffner, D. P., Cox, J. A., Rosenkrantz, J. G., and Richardson, W. R. (1979): Retroperitoneal lymph node dissection for Wilms tumor. *J. Pediatr. Surg.,* 14:704–707.

Rhabdomyosarcoma

Gilcksman, A. S., Maurer, H. M., and Vietti, T. J. (1979): Overview of conference on sarcomas of soft tissue and bone in childhood. *Med. Pediatr. Oncol.,* 7:55–67.

Kearney, M. M., Soule, E. H., and Ivins, J. C. (1980): Malignant fibrous histiocytoma. A retrospective study of 167 cases. *Cancer,* 45:167–178.

Neifeld, J. P., Maurer, H. M., Godwin, D., Berg, J. W., and Salzberg, A. M. (1979): Prognostic variables in pediatric rhabdomyosarcoma before and after multimodal therapy. *J. Pediatr. Surg.,* 14:699–703.

Ransom, J. L., Pratt, C. B., Hustu, H. O., Kumar, A. P. M., Howarth, C. B., and Bowles, D. (1980): Retroperitoneal rhabdomyosarcoma in children. Results of multimodality therapy. *Cancer,* 45:845–850.

Ewing's Sarcoma

Glicksman, A. A., Maurer, H. M., and Vietti, T. J. (1979): Overview of conference on sarcomas of soft tissue and bone in childhood. *Med. Pediatr. Oncol.,* 7:55–67.

Graham-Pole, J. (1978): Ewing's sarcoma: treatment with high-dose radiation and adjuvant chemotherapy. *Med. Pediatr. Oncol.,* 7:1–8.

Osteosarcoma

Carter, S. K. (1980): The dilemma of adjuvant chemotherapy for osteogenic sarcoma. *Cancer Clin. Trials,* 3:29–36.

Glicksman, A. A., Maurer, H. M., and Vietti, T. J. (1979): Overview of conference on sarcomas of soft tissue and bone in childhood. *Med. Pediatr. Oncol.,* 7:55–67.

Wang, Y.-M., Sutow, W. W., Romsdahl, M. M., and Perez, C. (1979): Age-related pharmacokinetics of high-dose methotrexate in patients with osteosarcoma. *Cancer Treat. Rep.,* 63:405–410.

Cost of Survival

Cairns, N. U., Clark, G. M., Smith, S. D., and Lansky, S. B. (1979): Adaptation of siblings to childhood malignancy. *J. Pediatr.,* 95:484–487.

Deasy-Spinetta, P., and Spinetta, J. J. (1979): The child with cancer in school. Teachers' appraisal. *Am. J. Hematol. Oncol.,* 2:89–94.

Green, M. H., Glaubiger, D. L., Mead, G. D., and Joseph, F. (1979): Subsequent cancer in patients with Ewings' sarcoma. *Cancer Treat. Rep.,* 63:2043–2046.

Kinlein, L. J., Sheil, A. G. R., Peto, J., and Doll, R. (1979): Collaborative United Kingdom—Austrasian study of cancer in patients treated with immunosuppressive drugs. *Br. Med. J.,* 2:1461–1466.

Shimaoka, K., Getaz, E. P., Razack, M., Rao, U., Norman, M., Wallace, H. J., Jr., Shedd, D. P., and Walsh, D. (1979): Thyroid screening program for irradiated population. *NY State J. Med.,* 79:1525–1527.

Subject Index

A

Actinomycin D (AMD),
  57, 201
Adriamycin (ADR), 57
Age
  distribution
    of childhood tumors, 3, 5-6
    of Ewing's sarcoma, 150-151
    of neuroblastoma, 81-84
    of osteosarcoma, 171
    of rhabdomyosarcoma, 136
    of Wilms' tumor, 107-108,
      118-119
  radiation-induced tumors and,
    200
  survival relation to
    in childhood tumors, 6-7
    in neuroblastoma, 37, 75,
      81, 92-95
    in Wilms' tumor, 37, 115
Amputation
  for Ewing's sarcoma, 154-156
  for osteosarcoma, 178-179
Angiosarcoma, vinyl chloride
    and, 11
Aniridia, Wilms' tumor and,
    108, 118
Asbestos, pleural mesothelioma
    and, 11

B

1,3-bis(B-chloroethyl)-1-nitros-
    ourea (BCNU), 57
Bleomycin, 57
Bone
  metastases to, 37, 180-181
  tumors, 3

Brain tumors
  chemotherapy for, 64-65, 67
  multimodal therapy in, 50
Breast cancer, 9, 212

C

Cancer(s)
  of childhood, see Malignant
    solid tumors, of childhood
  familial, 10, 13, 212
  hereditary, 12, 118
  population at risk for, 10
  radiation-induced, 11, 165-
    166, 200-201
  relative frequencies of, in adults
    and children, 7-9
Carcinogenesis, see Oncogenesis
Carcinogenic hazards, of chemo-
    therapeutic agents, 13, 201
Carcinogens, 11
Carcinomas, in childhood, 8-9, 11,
    62
Cardiomyopathy, chemotherapeutic
    agents and, 56-57, 61
Carmustine, 57
Central nervous system, tumors of,
    5, 9, 37
Cervix, clear cell carcinoma of,
    11
Chemotherapeutic agents, 55-59
  abbreviations used for, 55
  carcinogenic hazards of, 13, 201
  caution with, 56-58
  route of administration of, 56-58
  therapeutic dose for, 56-58
  toxicity of, 56-58
Chemotherapy, 53-67